Into the Depths of the Mind: Exploring Mysterious 25 BRAIN Disorders

Erkan YILDIRIM

A Journey Through the Labyrinths of the Least Understood Neurological Conditions

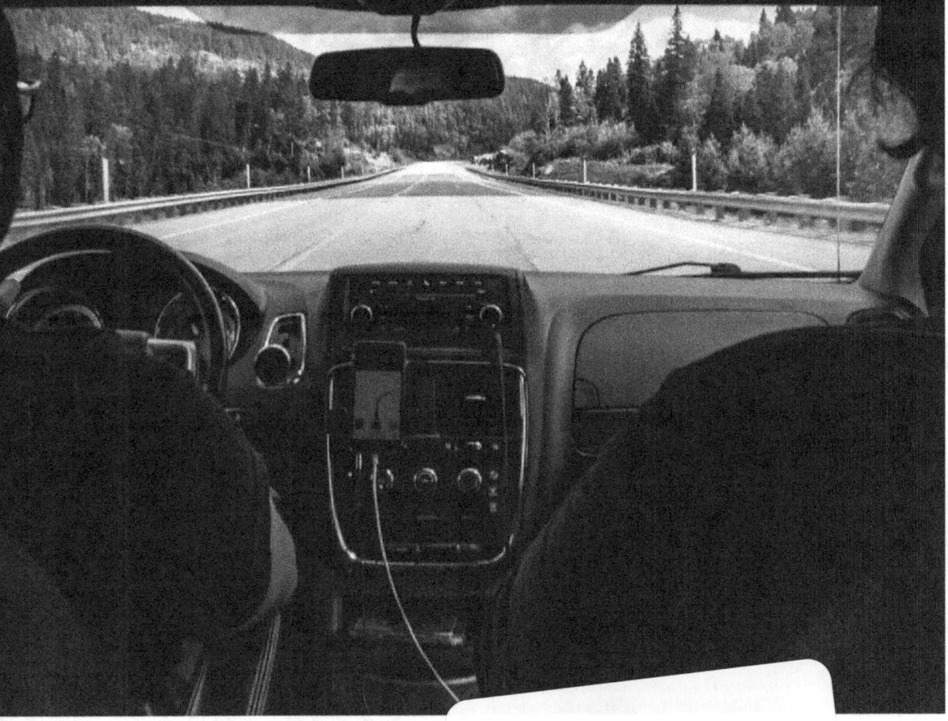

Table Of Contents

Note: This book is intended to provide a comprehensive overview
of rare and mysterious brain disorders, featuring case studies,
diagnostic criteria, treatment options, and personal stories. It is
designed to be accessible to a wide range of audiences, from
medical professionals to patients and caregivers, as well as those
with a general interest in neuroscience and rare diseases.

01

Chapter 1: Introduction to Rare Brain Disorders

Defining Rare Brain Disorders

In the subchapter "Defining Rare Brain Disorders," we delve into the complex world of neurological conditions that are not commonly seen in medical practice. These disorders, often referred to as rare diseases, present unique challenges for healthcare professionals in terms of diagnosis, treatment, and management.
Rare brain disorders encompass a wide range of conditions that affect the brain and nervous system, leading to a variety of symptoms and complications. These disorders can be genetic, acquired, or of unknown origin, making them particularly challenging to study and understand.

Medical professionals and students in the fields of neurology, psychiatry, general medicine, nursing, and other healthcare specialties may encounter patients with rare brain disorders throughout their careers. By expanding their knowledge and understanding of these conditions, they can better serve their patients and provide optimal care.

Academics and researchers involved in neuroscience, psychology, or neurological research can also benefit from studying rare brain disorders. These conditions offer unique insights into the inner workings of the brain and can provide valuable information for advancing scientific knowledge and developing new treatments.

For patients and caregivers affected by rare brain disorders, this subchapter offers detailed information and personal stories that may provide insights and support. Advocacy groups and non-governmental organizations dedicated to supporting individuals with rare diseases can also use this book as an educational resource to inform their work and raise awareness in their communities.

Ultimately, "Defining Rare Brain Disorders" serves as a valuable resource for a diverse audience, including healthcare professionals, researchers, patients, caregivers, advocacy groups, and individuals with a general interest in health and medicine. By exploring the mysteries of these conditions, we can deepen our understanding of the human brain and work towards improving outcomes for those affected by rare brain disorders.

The study of rare brain disorders holds immense importance in the field of medicine and neuroscience. While common neurological conditions like Alzheimer's and Parkinson's are well-known and extensively researched, rare brain disorders often present unique challenges and mysteries that can deepen our understanding of the complexities of the human brain.

For medical professionals and students, delving into the world of rare brain disorders can provide invaluable insights into the intricacies of brain function and pathology. By studying these less-common conditions, neurologists, psychiatrists, general physicians, nurses, and medical students can expand their knowledge base and develop more effective treatment strategies for their patients.

Academics and researchers in the fields of neuroscience and psychology can also benefit from exploring rare brain disorders. These conditions offer a wealth of research opportunities that can lead to groundbreaking discoveries and advancements in the field of brain science.

Patients, caregivers, advocacy groups, and NGOs dedicated to rare brain disorders can find valuable information and support in a comprehensive resource like "Into the Depths of the Mind." By understanding the symptoms, causes, and treatment options for these conditions, individuals and organizations can better advocate for improved care and support for those affected by rare brain disorders. Even for health enthusiasts, lifelong learners, and non-specialists, the exploration of rare brain disorders can be a fascinating journey into the depths of the human mind. By delving into the stories and science behind these mysterious conditions, readers can gain a deeper appreciation for the complexity and resilience of the human brain.

Overview of the Book

Importance of Studying Rare Brain Disorders

Health enthusiasts, curious minds, and non-specialists with an interest in medicine and rare diseases will be captivated by the fascinating stories and insights shared in this book. From the intricacies of the human brain to the mysteries of rare neurological conditions, "Into the Depths of the Mind" offers a compelling journey into the depths of the human mind."

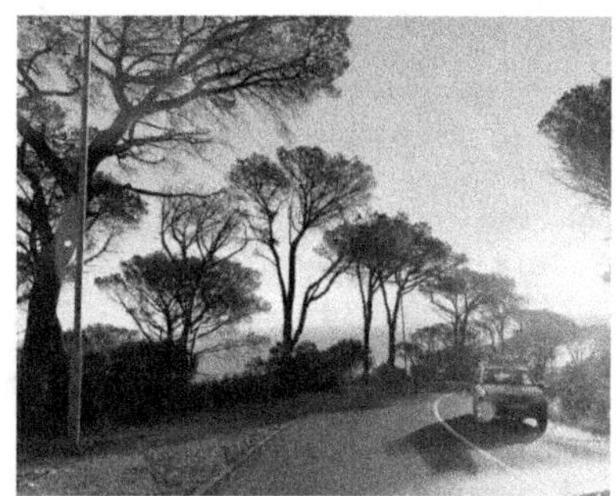

"Into the Depths of the Mind: Exploring Mysterious Brain Disorders" delves into the intriguing world of rare and mysterious brain disorders, offering a comprehensive overview of 25 lesser-known conditions that challenge our understanding of the human mind. This book is designed to serve as a valuable resource for a diverse audience, including medical professionals, researchers, patients and caregivers, advocacy groups, health enthusiasts, and lifelong learners.

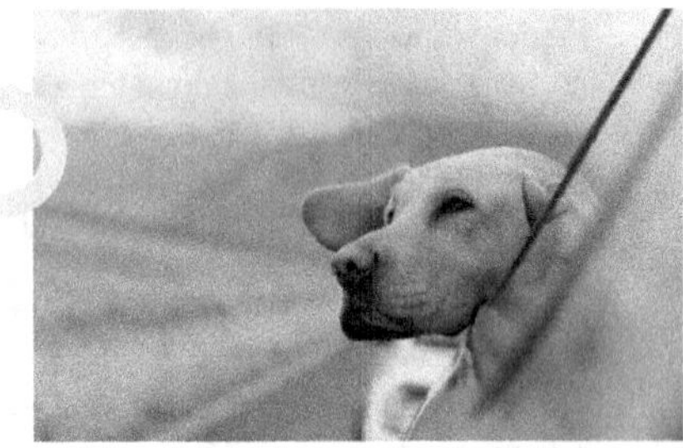

For medical professionals and students in the fields of neurology, psychiatry, general medicine, nursing, and healthcare, this book provides in-depth information on a variety of brain disorders that may not be commonly encountered in clinical practice. By expanding their knowledge and awareness of these conditions, healthcare professionals can better serve their patients and contribute to advancements in the field of neuroscience.

Academics and researchers will find this collection of rare diseases to be a valuable reference for their studies and research endeavors. The detailed insights and case studies presented in the book can enhance their understanding of complex neurological disorders and inspire new avenues of research.

Patients, caregivers, and advocacy groups dedicated to supporting individuals with rare brain disorders will appreciate the personal stories and detailed information provided in the book. By gaining a deeper understanding of these conditions, they can find solace, support, and valuable resources to navigate the challenges they may face.

Creutzfeldt-Jakob Disease

Creutzfeldt-Jakob Disease (CJD) is a rare and fatal neurodegenerative disorder that affects the brain, causing rapid cognitive decline, movement disorders, and eventually leading to death. This mysterious disease is caused by abnormal prion proteins that multiply and spread throughout the brain, causing damage to nerve cells.

Medical professionals and students, especially neurologists and psychiatrists, need to be aware of CJD due to its unique characteristics and devastating impact on patients. General physicians and nurses may encounter patients with CJD symptoms and must understand the importance of early diagnosis and management.

Researchers and academics in the field of neuroscience and psychology can benefit from studying CJD to unravel its underlying mechanisms and potential treatment options. Medical libraries and institutions may consider adding resources on CJD to support students and researchers in their quest for knowledge.

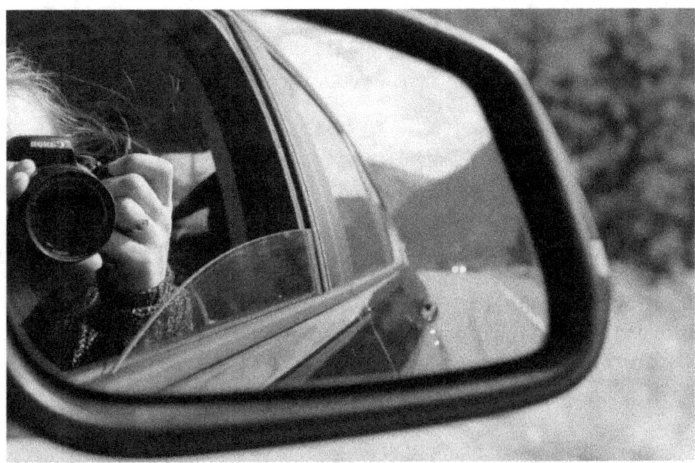

For patients and caregivers dealing with a CJD diagnosis, understanding the disease's progression and potential challenges is crucial for providing effective care and support. Advocacy groups and NGOs focused on rare brain disorders can use this information to educate their communities and advocate for better resources and support. Health enthusiasts and lifelong learners interested in delving into the complexities of rare diseases like CJD will find valuable insights in exploring the depths of the mind through this book. Non-specialists with a curiosity for the mysteries of the human body will also find this subchapter on CJD a fascinating read, shedding light on one of the lesser-known brain disorders.

Huntington's Disease

Huntington's Disease, also known as Huntington's chorea, is a devastating neurological disorder that impacts both the body and mind. This genetic disorder is caused by a mutation in the huntingtin gene, leading to the degeneration of nerve cells in the brain. Patients with Huntington's Disease often experience involuntary movements, cognitive decline, and psychiatric symptoms.
For medical professionals and students, understanding Huntington's Disease is crucial for early detection and intervention. Neurologists and psychiatrists may encounter patients with this disorder and need to provide appropriate care and support. General physicians and nurses may also come across individuals with Huntington's Disease in their practice and should be equipped with knowledge on how to manage the symptoms effectively.

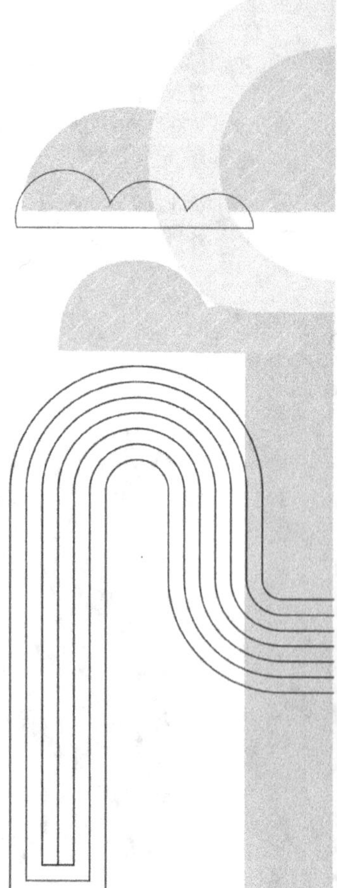

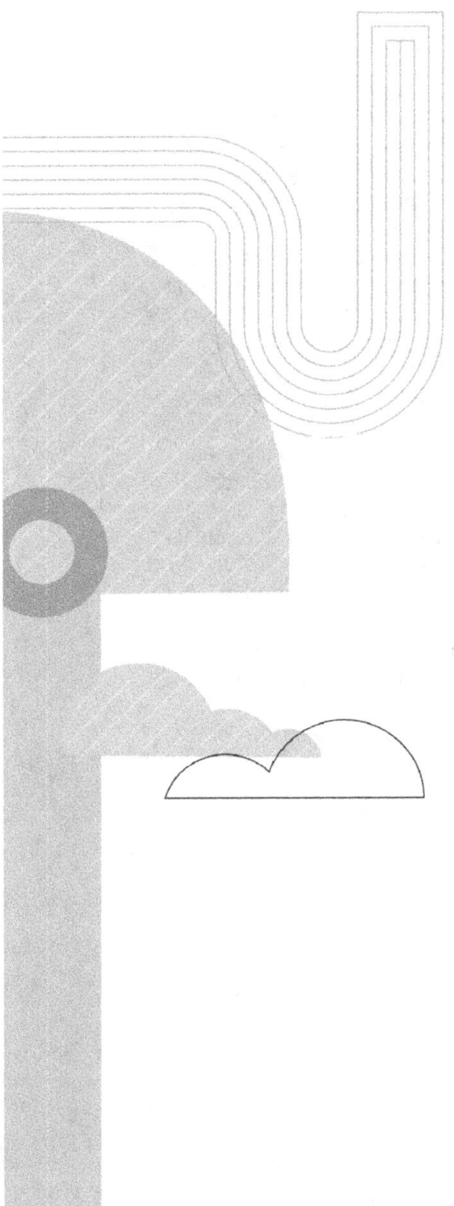

Researchers and academics in the field of neuroscience and psychology can benefit from studying Huntington's Disease to further explore the complexities of the human brain. By delving into the mechanisms behind this disorder, new insights and potential treatment options may be discovered. Patients and caregivers affected by Huntington's Disease may find solace in learning more about their condition through the book. Personal stories and detailed information can offer support and guidance on how to cope with the challenges that come with this rare disease.

Advocacy groups and NGOs dedicated to supporting individuals with rare brain disorders can utilize the book as an educational resource to raise awareness and promote understanding within their communities.

Health enthusiasts, lifelong learners, and non-specialists interested in the mysteries of the human body may also find the chapter on Huntington's Disease to be a fascinating read. Exploring the depths of this rare neurological disorder can provide a deeper understanding of the complexities of the brain and the impact it has on one's quality of life.

Progressive Supranuclear Palsy

Progressive Supranuclear Palsy (PSP) is a rare neurological disorder that affects movement, balance, vision, speech, and cognition. This subchapter delves into the intricacies of this enigmatic condition, providing valuable insights for medical professionals and students seeking to broaden their understanding of less-common brain disorders.

Neurologists, psychiatrists, general physicians, nurses, and medical students will find detailed information on the clinical presentation, diagnostic criteria, and management strategies for patients with PSP. By exploring the unique challenges faced by individuals with this condition, healthcare professionals can enhance their ability to provide comprehensive care and support to those affected by PSP.

Academics and researchers involved in neuroscience, psychology, or neurological research will find this subchapter to be a valuable resource for academic and research purposes. By delving into the latest advancements in PSP research, scholars can contribute to the growing body of knowledge surrounding this complex disorder.

Patients, caregivers, advocacy groups, and NGOs dedicated to supporting individuals with rare brain disorders will benefit from the detailed information and personal stories shared in this subchapter. By gaining a deeper understanding of PSP, individuals and organizations can advocate for improved care, resources, and support for those living with this challenging condition.

Health enthusiasts, lifelong learners, and non-specialists with a curiosity for the mysteries of the human body will also find this subchapter to be a fascinating exploration of Progressive Supranuclear Palsy. By delving into the depths of this rare disorder, readers can expand their knowledge and gain a deeper appreciation for the complexities of the human brain.

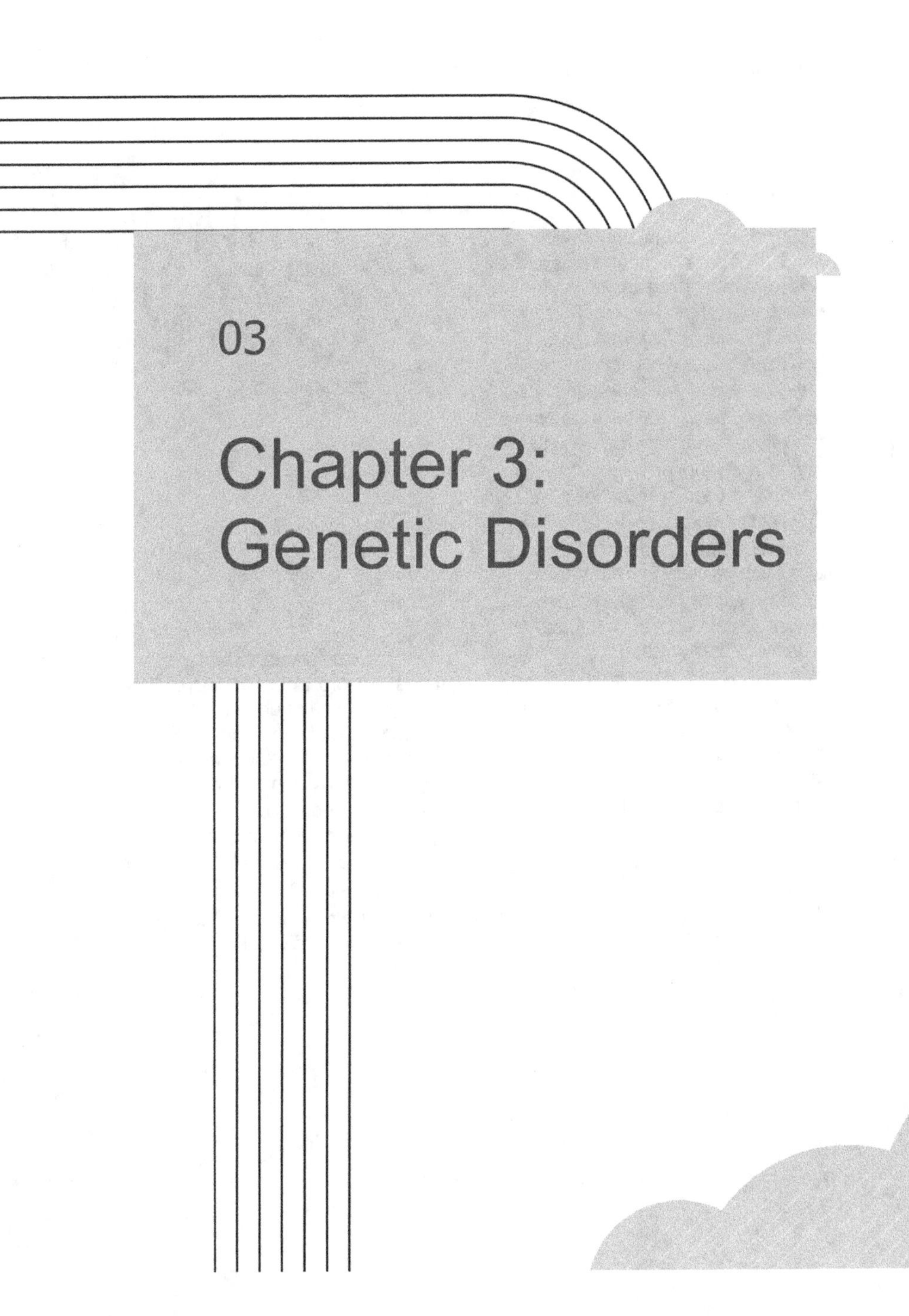

Chapter 3: Genetic Disorders

Rett Syndrome

Rett Syndrome is a rare neurological disorder that primarily affects girls and is characterized by a regression in development after a period of normal growth. Individuals with Rett Syndrome often experience a loss of purposeful hand skills, language abilities, and motor coordination, as well as the development of repetitive hand movements such as wringing, clapping, or tapping. This disorder is caused by mutations in the MECP2 gene, which plays a crucial role in brain development and function. Medical professionals and students, especially neurologists and psychiatrists, may encounter patients with Rett Syndrome in their practice and should be familiar with the symptoms and management of this condition. Nurses and general physicians may also benefit from understanding the unique challenges faced by individuals with Rett Syndrome and their families.

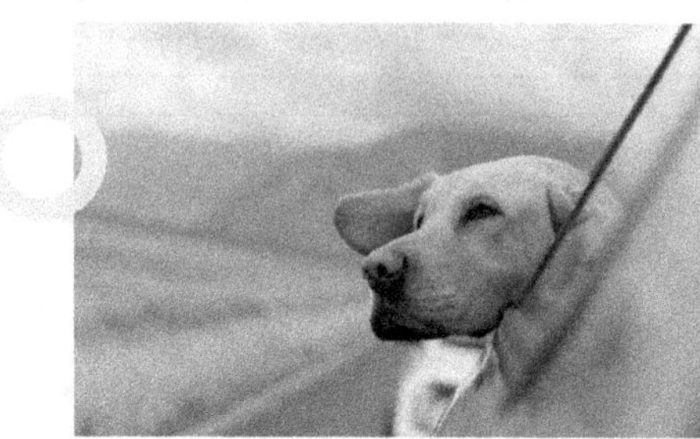

Researchers and academics in the fields of neuroscience and psychology can delve into the underlying mechanisms of Rett Syndrome and explore potential treatments or interventions to improve the quality of life for affected individuals. Medical librarians and institutions can provide access to resources like "Minds on the Brink: Unveiling 25 Rare and Mysterious Brain Disorders" to support students and researchers in their studies.

Patients, caregivers, advocacy groups, and health enthusiasts seeking information on Rett Syndrome may find valuable insights and support in this book. By shedding light on lesser-known neurological disorders like Rett Syndrome, we can enhance our understanding of the human brain and work towards better outcomes for those affected by these conditions.

Angelman Syndrome

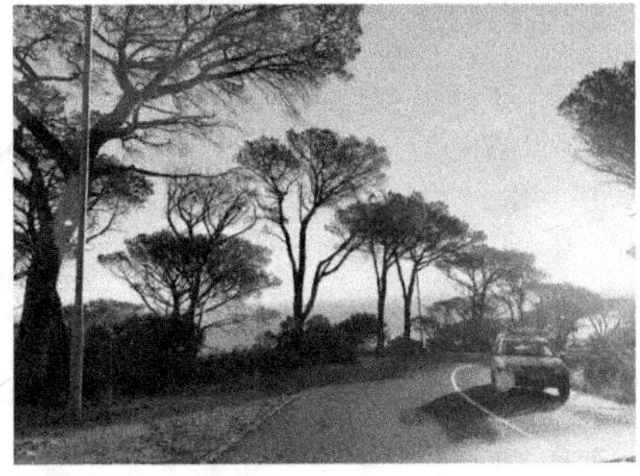

Angelman Syndrome is a rare genetic disorder that affects the nervous system, causing developmental delays, speech impairments, and movement disorders. Individuals with Angelman Syndrome often exhibit a happy demeanor, with frequent laughter and smiling. However, they may also experience seizures, sleep disturbances, and difficulty with balance and coordination.

Medical professionals and students, particularly neurologists, psychiatrists, general physicians, nurses, and medical students, will find valuable information on the diagnosis and management of Angelman Syndrome in this subchapter. Understanding the underlying genetic causes and associated symptoms can aid in providing effective care and support for patients with this condition.

Academics and researchers interested in neuroscience, psychology, or neurological research will benefit from exploring the complexities of Angelman Syndrome. By delving into the molecular mechanisms and brain abnormalities associated with this disorder, new insights and potential treatment strategies may be uncovered.

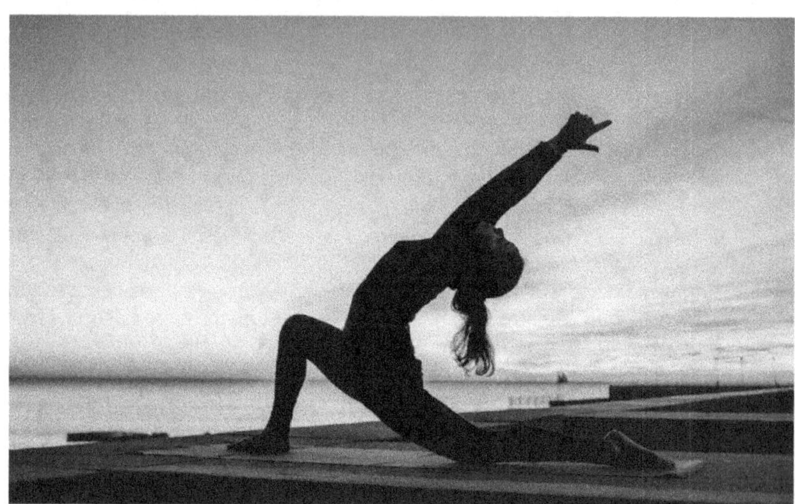

Patients, caregivers, and advocacy groups dedicated to supporting individuals with rare brain disorders can gain valuable knowledge and resources from this subchapter. Personal stories and experiences shared within the book can provide a sense of community and understanding for those living with Angelman Syndrome.
Health enthusiasts, lifelong learners, and non-specialists with a curiosity for the mysteries of the human brain will find this subchapter to be an enlightening and informative read. By expanding their knowledge of less-common neurological disorders like Angelman Syndrome, readers can deepen their understanding of the intricacies of the mind and body.

Fragile X Syndrome

Fragile X Syndrome is a genetic condition that causes a range of developmental problems, including learning disabilities and cognitive impairment. It is the most common inherited cause of intellectual disability in males and a significant cause of intellectual disability in females. This syndrome is caused by a mutation in the FMR1 gene on the X chromosome, which leads to a lack of production of a protein essential for brain development.

Individuals with Fragile X Syndrome may exhibit a variety of symptoms, including social and communication difficulties, hyperactivity, repetitive behaviors, and sensory sensitivities. They may also have physical features such as a long face, large ears, and a prominent jaw. Early intervention and support are crucial in helping individuals with Fragile X Syndrome reach their full potential.

Diagnosing Fragile X Syndrome involves genetic testing to identify the gene mutation. Treatment typically involves a multidisciplinary approach, including speech therapy, occupational therapy, behavioral therapy, and educational interventions. Medications may also be prescribed to manage symptoms such as anxiety and hyperactivity.

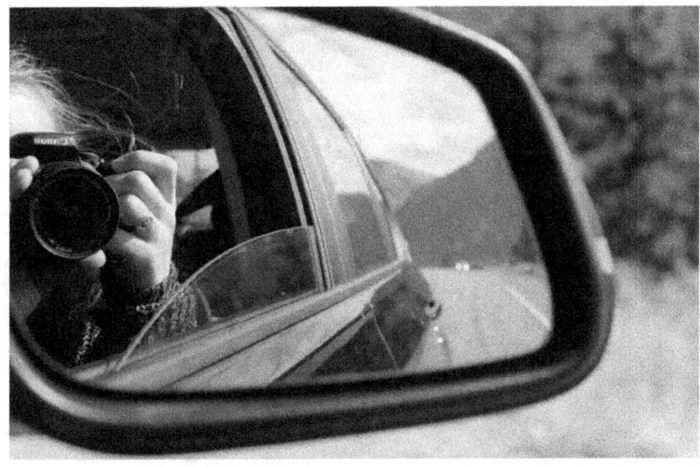

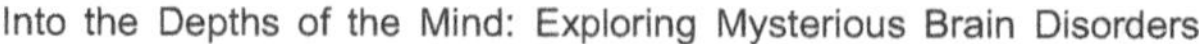

As medical professionals and researchers, understanding Fragile X Syndrome is essential for providing accurate diagnoses and effective treatments. By delving into the complexities of this disorder, we can better support patients and their families in navigating the challenges they may face. Through ongoing research and advancements in treatment options, we can continue to improve the quality of life for individuals with Fragile X Syndrome.

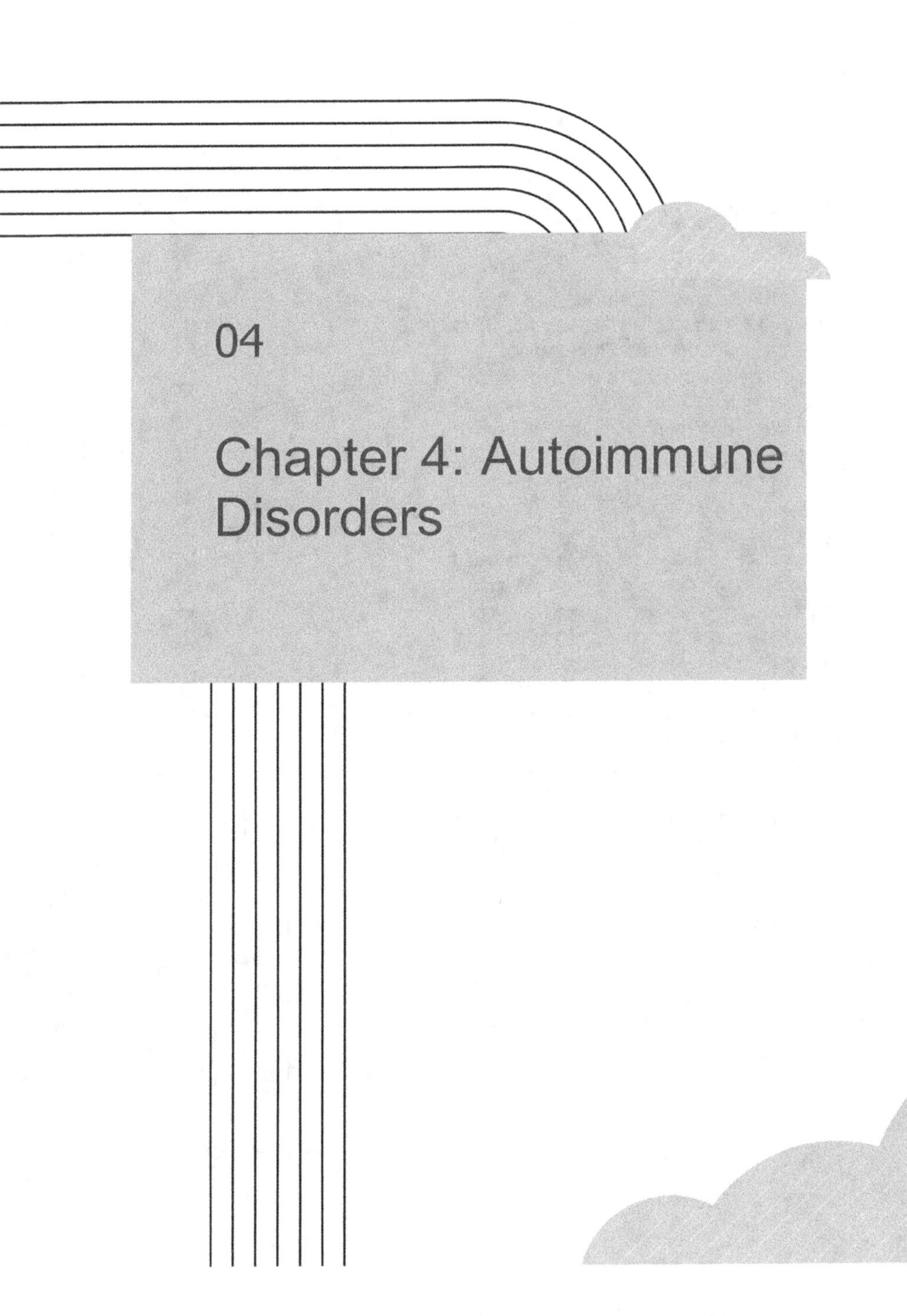

04

Chapter 4: Autoimmune Disorders

Anti-NMDA Receptor Encephalitis

Anti-NMDA Receptor Encephalitis is a rare and complex brain disorder that falls under the umbrella of autoimmune encephalitis. This condition is characterized by the body's immune system mistakenly attacking the NMDA receptors in the brain, leading to a range of neurological and psychiatric symptoms.

Medical professionals and students in neurology, psychiatry, and general medicine may encounter patients with Anti-NMDA Receptor Encephalitis in their practice, making it crucial to understand the intricacies of this disorder. Nurses and other healthcare professionals may also benefit from learning about the symptoms, diagnosis, and treatment options for this condition to provide comprehensive care to affected individuals.

For researchers and academics in neuroscience and psychology, studying Anti-NMDA Receptor Encephalitis can provide valuable insights into the interplay between the immune system and the brain. By delving into the mechanisms underlying this disorder, researchers can contribute to the development of more effective treatment strategies and potentially uncover new avenues for therapeutic interventions.

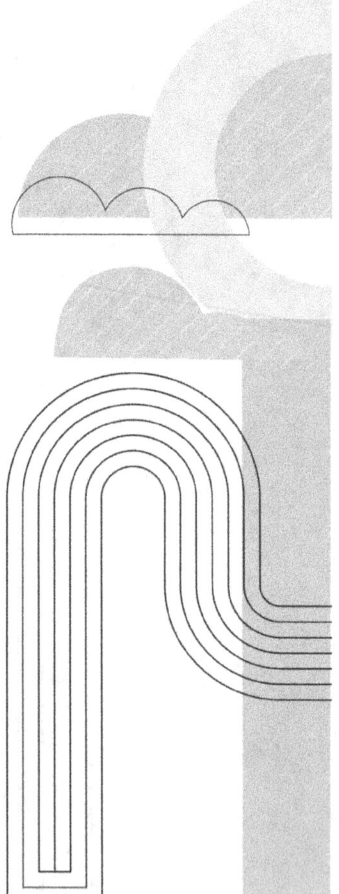

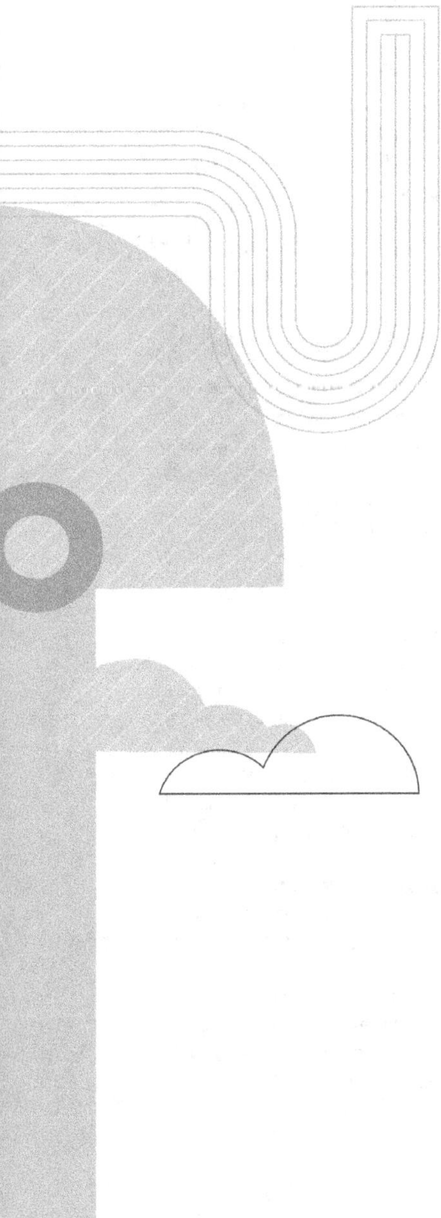

Patients diagnosed with Anti-NMDA Receptor Encephalitis, as well as their families and caregivers, may find solace in understanding the nature of their condition and the available treatment options. Personal stories and experiences shared in the book can offer emotional support and guidance to those navigating the challenges of living with this rare brain disorder.

Ultimately, "Into the Depths of the Mind: Exploring Mysterious Brain Disorders" serves as a valuable resource for a diverse audience, from medical professionals and researchers to patients, caregivers, and health enthusiasts. By shedding light on lesser-known conditions like Anti-NMDA Receptor Encephalitis, the book aims to broaden understanding and foster empathy towards individuals affected by these mysterious disorders.

Stiff Person Syndrome

Stiff Person Syndrome (SPS) is a rare neurological disorder characterized by debilitating muscle stiffness and spasms, often triggered by emotional distress or sudden movements. This condition, though uncommon, can have a significant impact on the quality of life for those affected.

Patients with Stiff Person Syndrome may experience episodes of severe muscle rigidity, commonly affecting the trunk and limbs, making movement difficult and painful. These episodes can be so severe that individuals may become completely immobile, leading to challenges in daily activities and independence.

The exact cause of SPS is not fully understood, but it is believed to involve an autoimmune response targeting the nervous system. This autoimmune attack leads to the destruction of inhibitory neurons responsible for regulating muscle tone, resulting in the characteristic stiffness and spasms seen in SPS patients.

Diagnosis of Stiff Person Syndrome can be challenging due to its rarity and similarity to other neurological conditions. A comprehensive evaluation, including clinical symptoms, imaging studies, and laboratory tests, is crucial for accurate diagnosis and appropriate management.

Treatment for SPS typically involves a combination of medications to reduce muscle stiffness and spasms, along with physical therapy to improve mobility and function. In some cases, intravenous immunoglobulin therapy or plasma exchange may be considered to modulate the immune response and alleviate symptoms.

As medical professionals, it is essential to be aware of rare disorders like Stiff Person Syndrome to provide timely and effective care for patients presenting with unusual symptoms. By expanding our understanding of these mysterious brain disorders, we can offer better support and treatment options for those in need.

Neuromyelitis Optica

Neuromyelitis Optica, also known as Devic's disease, is a rare autoimmune disorder that affects the optic nerves and spinal cord. This condition is characterized by inflammation and damage to the myelin sheath, the protective covering of nerve fibers. As a result, individuals with neuromyelitis optica may experience vision loss, weakness, paralysis, and sensory disturbances.

One of the hallmark features of neuromyelitis optica is the presence of specific antibodies called aquaporin-4 antibodies. These antibodies target a protein found in the cells of the central nervous system, leading to the immune system attacking the optic nerves and spinal cord.

Diagnosing neuromyelitis optica can be challenging due to its similarity to other neurological conditions, such as multiple sclerosis. However, advanced imaging techniques, spinal fluid analysis, and antibody testing can help differentiate between these disorders.

Treatment for neuromyelitis optica typically involves managing symptoms, preventing relapses, and preserving neurological function. Immunosuppressive medications, corticosteroids, plasma exchange, and physical therapy are commonly used to help patients manage their symptoms and improve their quality of life.

Research into neuromyelitis optica is ongoing, with a focus on understanding the underlying mechanisms of the disease and developing targeted therapies. By raising awareness of this rare neurological disorder, healthcare professionals can better support patients, improve diagnostic accuracy, and enhance treatment outcomes.

05

Chapter 5:
Infectious Disorders

Neurocysticercosis

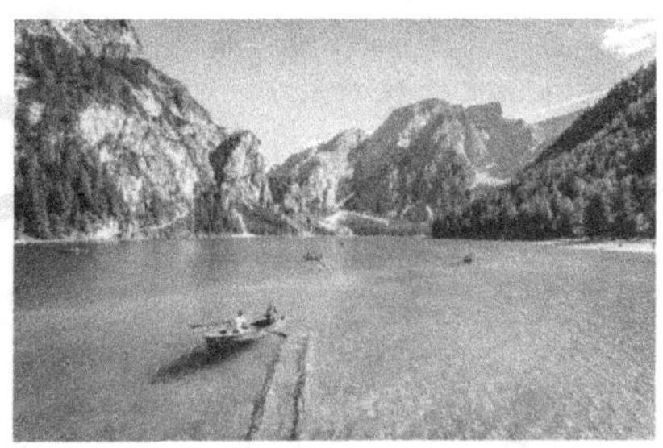

Neurocysticercosis is a parasitic infection of the central nervous system caused by the larvae of the tapeworm Taenia solium. This condition is prevalent in regions where pork is consumed and sanitation practices are poor. The larvae can invade the brain, spinal cord, or other tissues, leading to a range of neurological symptoms.

For medical professionals and students, understanding neurocysticercosis is crucial in regions where this disease is endemic. Neurologists, psychiatrists, general physicians, nurses, and medical students must be able to recognize the symptoms of this condition and provide appropriate treatment. By delving into the depths of this mysterious brain disorder, healthcare professionals can broaden their expertise and improve patient care. Academics and researchers interested in neuroscience or neurological research can benefit from studying neurocysticercosis to expand their knowledge of rare brain disorders. By exploring the complexities of this condition, researchers may uncover new insights into the pathophysiology and treatment options for neurocysticercosis.

Patients, caregivers, advocacy groups, and health enthusiasts can also find valuable information in this subchapter. Understanding the symptoms, diagnosis, and treatment of neurocysticercosis can provide support and guidance to individuals affected by this condition. Additionally, raising awareness of neurocysticercosis can help advocacy groups and NGOs in their efforts to support and educate communities impacted by this disease.

Overall, delving into the depths of neurocysticercosis can provide a comprehensive understanding of this rare and mysterious brain disorder for a diverse audience of healthcare professionals, researchers, patients, caregivers, and health enthusiasts.

Progressive Multifocal Leukoencephalopathy

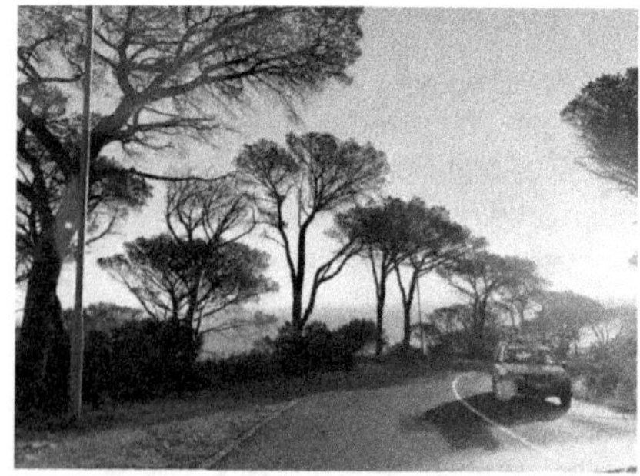

Progressive Multifocal Leukoencephalopathy (PML) is a rare and potentially fatal brain disorder that primarily affects individuals with weakened immune systems. This condition is caused by the JC virus, a common virus that is usually harmless but can become dangerous in individuals with compromised immune function. PML is characterized by the progressive damage to the white matter of the brain, leading to a range of symptoms such as weakness, cognitive impairment, vision problems, and difficulties with coordination.

Diagnosing PML can be challenging, as its symptoms can mimic those of other neurological conditions. Medical professionals should consider conducting brain imaging studies, cerebrospinal fluid analysis, and JC virus testing to confirm a PML diagnosis. Treatment options for PML are limited, and the focus is typically on managing symptoms and supporting the immune system.

As medical professionals and researchers, understanding PML is crucial for providing accurate diagnoses and appropriate care to patients. By delving into the depths of this mysterious brain disorder, we can expand our knowledge of how the JC virus interacts with the immune system and causes damage to the brain. Through research and collaboration, we can work towards developing more effective treatments and improving outcomes for individuals living with PML.

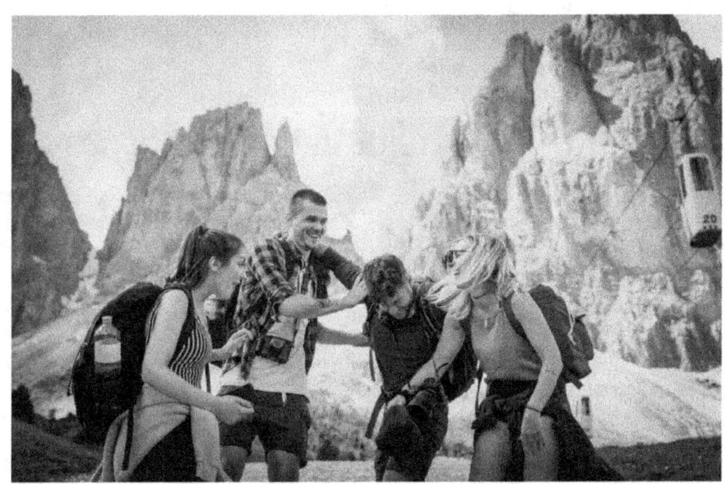

For patients, caregivers, and advocacy groups, having access to comprehensive information about PML can help in navigating the challenges of living with this condition. By sharing personal stories and insights, we can offer support and guidance to those affected by PML, fostering a sense of community and understanding.
Overall, exploring Progressive Multifocal Leukoencephalopathy sheds light on the complexities of the human brain and the devastating impact of neurological disorders on individuals and their loved ones. Through education, research, and advocacy, we can strive towards better outcomes and improved quality of life for those affected by PML.

Variant Creutzfeldt-Jakob Disease

Variant Creutzfeldt-Jakob Disease (vCJD) is a rare and fatal brain disorder that falls under the umbrella of prion diseases. This particular form of Creutzfeldt-Jakob Disease is unique as it is believed to be caused by the consumption of contaminated meat, specifically beef infected with the prion protein responsible for vCJD.

Symptoms of vCJD can include psychiatric symptoms such as depression, anxiety, and hallucinations, as well as neurological symptoms like muscle stiffness, loss of coordination, and cognitive decline. The disease progresses rapidly, leading to severe disability and ultimately death.

Diagnosis of vCJD can be challenging, as symptoms may mimic other neurological disorders. However, advanced imaging techniques and cerebrospinal fluid analysis can aid in confirming the presence of prions in the brain.

Treatment for vCJD is limited, with no cure currently available. Supportive care to manage symptoms and improve quality of life is typically the main focus of treatment.

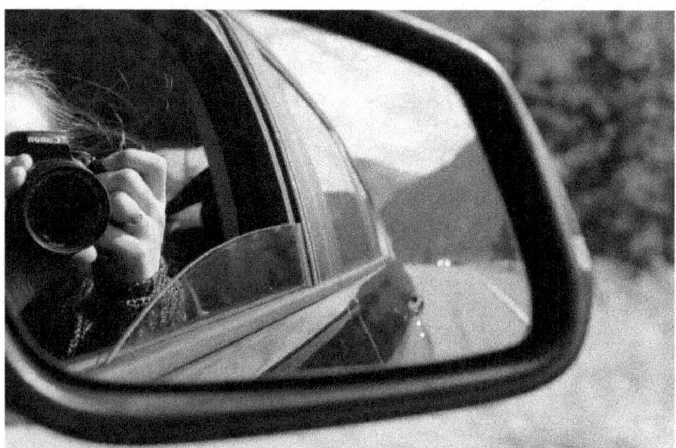

Medical professionals and researchers play a crucial role in understanding and studying vCJD to develop better diagnostic tools and potential treatments. Patients and caregivers affected by vCJD may find solace in connecting with advocacy groups and organizations dedicated to supporting individuals with rare brain disorders.

For those with a keen interest in exploring the depths of the human mind and its mysterious disorders, delving into the intricacies of vCJD can provide valuable insights into the complexities of the brain and the devastating impact of prion diseases.

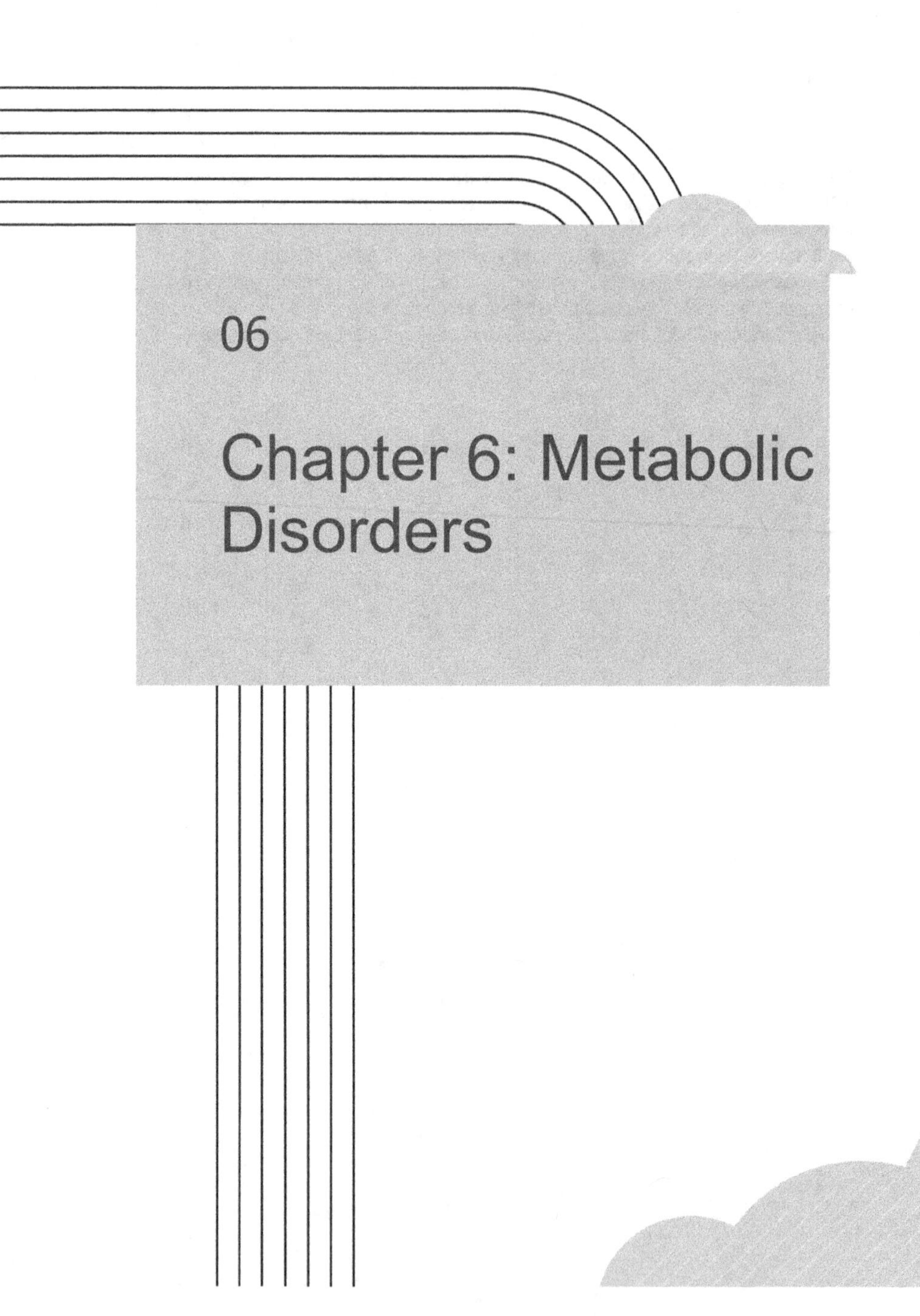

06

Chapter 6: Metabolic Disorders

Wilson's Disease

Wilson's disease is a rare genetic disorder that causes copper to accumulate in the body, particularly in the liver and brain. This build-up of copper can lead to a range of symptoms, including liver damage, neurological problems, and psychiatric disturbances. It is caused by mutations in the ATP7B gene, which is responsible for regulating copper levels in the body. Symptoms of Wilson's disease can vary widely and may include fatigue, jaundice, tremors, difficulty speaking or swallowing, personality changes, and even psychosis. Diagnosis can be challenging, as symptoms can mimic other conditions, but a combination of blood tests, imaging studies, and genetic testing can help confirm the presence of the disease.

Treatment for Wilson's disease involves reducing copper levels in the body through medications that bind to copper and help remove it from the system. In some cases, liver transplants may be necessary if the liver is severely damaged. It is crucial for patients with Wilson's disease to follow a strict treatment regimen and regularly monitor their copper levels to prevent complications.

For medical professionals and researchers, understanding Wilson's disease is essential for early detection and effective management. Patients and caregivers can benefit from detailed information on the disease, its symptoms, and treatment options. Advocacy groups and health enthusiasts can use this knowledge to raise awareness and support individuals affected by Wilson's disease.Overall, Wilson's disease serves as a reminder of the intricate relationship between genetics, metabolism, and brain health.

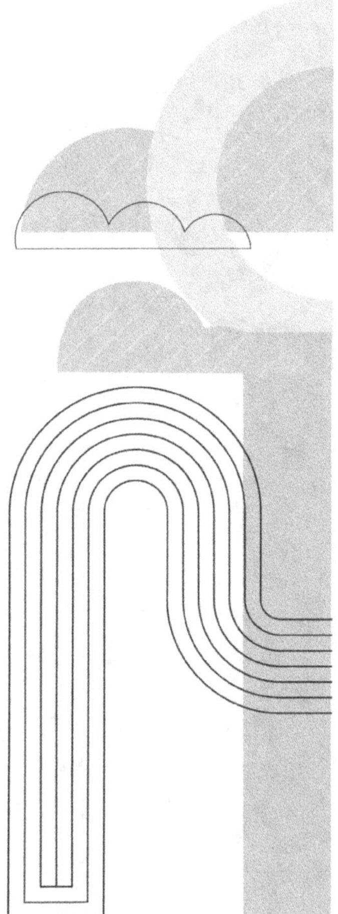

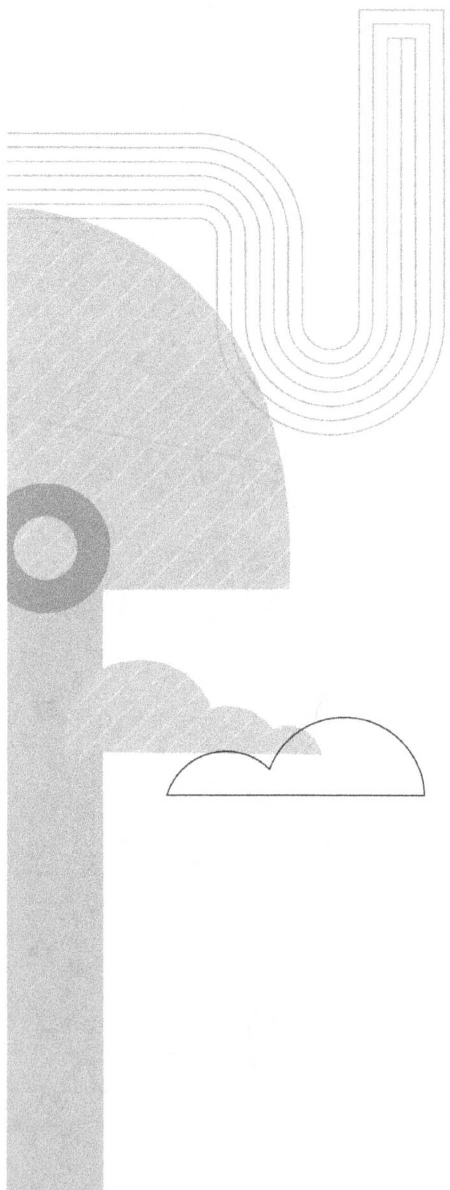

Maple Syrup Urine Disease

Maple Syrup Urine Disease (MSUD) is a rare genetic disorder that affects the body's ability to break down certain amino acids found in protein-rich foods. This results in a build-up of toxic substances in the blood and urine, giving off a distinct sweet smell reminiscent of maple syrup.

Medical professionals and students, especially those specializing in neurology, psychiatry, or general medicine, may encounter patients with MSUD in their practice. Understanding the intricacies of this disorder is crucial for accurate diagnosis and appropriate treatment.

Academics and researchers in the fields of neuroscience and psychology may find MSUD to be an intriguing subject for further study. By delving into the underlying mechanisms of this disorder, new insights into brain function and metabolism may be gained.

For patients and caregivers dealing with the challenges of MSUD, this subchapter provides valuable information on symptoms, management strategies, and support resources. Advocacy groups and NGOs dedicated to rare brain disorders can also benefit from the detailed explanations and personal stories shared in this book.

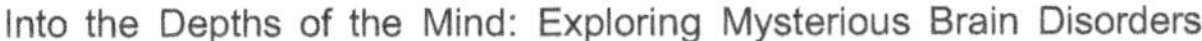

Health enthusiasts, lifelong learners, and non-specialists interested in exploring the mysteries of the human brain will find the discussion on MSUD to be both informative and enlightening. By shedding light on lesser-known disorders like MSUD, this book aims to broaden understanding and awareness of the complexities of the mind.

Adrenoleukodystrophy

Adrenoleukodystrophy, often referred to as ALD, is a rare and progressive genetic disorder that affects the nervous system and adrenal glands. This disorder is caused by a mutation in the ABCD1 gene, which leads to the accumulation of very long-chain fatty acids in the brain, spinal cord, and adrenal glands.

ALD primarily affects males, although females can also be carriers of the gene mutation. Symptoms of ALD typically appear in childhood, with the most severe form known as childhood cerebral ALD. This form of the disease progresses rapidly, leading to loss of cognitive and motor function, as well as behavioral changes.

Another form of ALD is adrenomyeloneuropathy, which primarily affects adult males. This form of the disease is characterized by weakness in the legs, bladder and bowel dysfunction, and peripheral neuropathy.

Diagnosis of ALD is typically confirmed through genetic testing and imaging studies such as MRI. Treatment options for ALD are limited, and currently, the most effective intervention is stem cell transplantation, which can slow the progression of the disease if performed early in childhood cerebral ALD.

As medical professionals and researchers, it is crucial to understand the complexities of Adrenoleukodystrophy to provide accurate diagnosis and appropriate care for patients. By delving into the depths of this mysterious brain disorder, we can work towards improving the quality of life for individuals affected by ALD and their families.

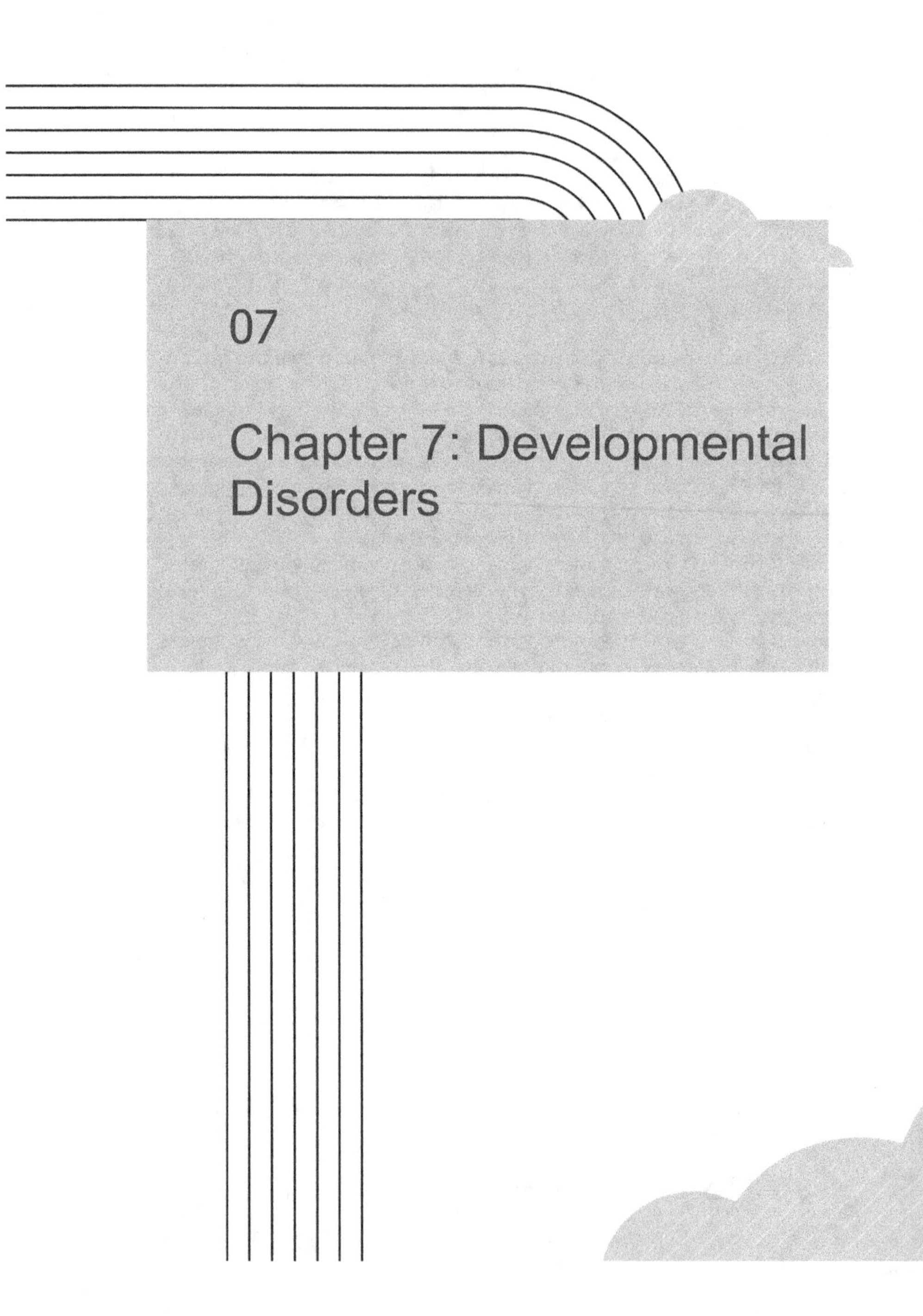

Chapter 7: Developmental Disorders

Agenesis of the Corpus Callosum

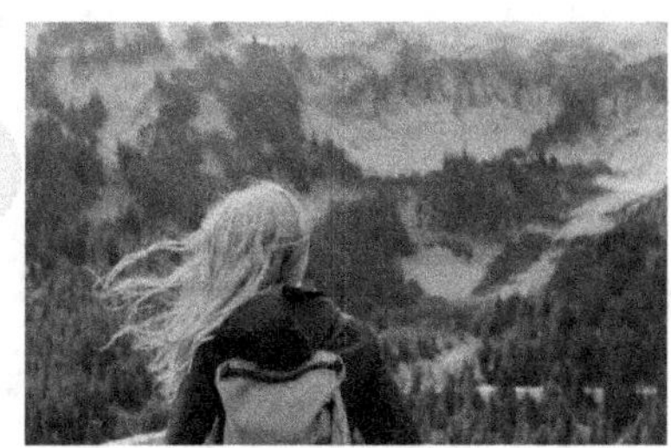

Agenesis of the corpus callosum is a rare neurological condition where an individual is born without a corpus callosum, the structure that connects the two hemispheres of the brain. This results in a range of neurological symptoms and challenges for those affected.

In this subchapter, we delve into the intricacies of this mysterious disorder, exploring its causes, symptoms, diagnosis, and potential treatments. Medical professionals and students, particularly neurologists, psychiatrists, general physicians, nurses, and medical students, will find this information invaluable for understanding and identifying this rare condition in their patients.

Academics and researchers in the fields of neuroscience, psychology, and neurology will benefit from the detailed insights provided in this chapter, which can serve as a valuable resource for academic and research purposes. Medical libraries and institutions may also find this book to be a valuable addition to their collections, providing students and researchers with a comprehensive understanding of less-common neurological disorders.

Patients diagnosed with agenesis of the corpus callosum, as well as their families and caregivers, can gain valuable information and insights from this subchapter, helping them navigate the challenges associated with this condition. Advocacy groups and NGOs dedicated to supporting individuals with rare brain disorders can also use this book as an educational resource to further their work and share knowledge within their communities.

For health enthusiasts, lifelong learners, and non-specialists with a curiosity for the mysteries of the human brain, this subchapter offers a fascinating exploration into a little-known disorder, expanding their knowledge and understanding of the complexities of the mind.

Chiari Malformation

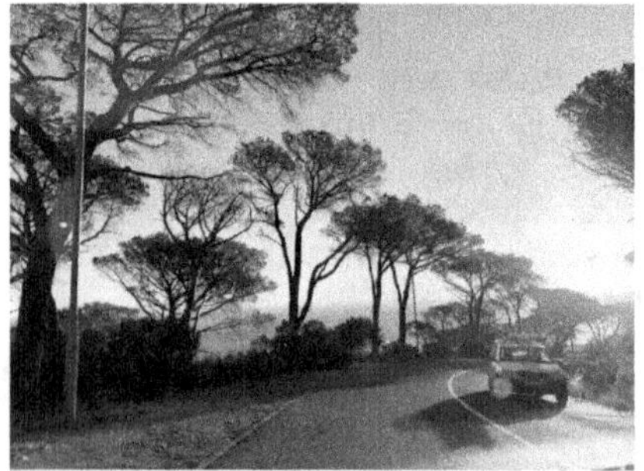

Chiari Malformation is a neurological condition in which the lower part of the brain, known as the cerebellum, extends into the spinal canal. This displacement can put pressure on the brain and spinal cord, leading to a range of symptoms such as headaches, neck pain, balance problems, and muscle weakness.

There are several types of Chiari Malformation, with Type I being the most common. This type is often present from birth but may not cause symptoms until later in life. Type II and Type III are more severe forms of the condition and are typically diagnosed in infancy or childhood.

Diagnosis of Chiari Malformation usually involves a combination of imaging tests such as MRI or CT scans, along with a thorough physical examination. Treatment options vary depending on the severity of symptoms and may include medication for pain management, physical therapy, or in some cases, surgery to alleviate pressure on the brain and spinal cord.

For medical professionals and students, understanding Chiari Malformation is crucial for accurately diagnosing and treating patients who present with these symptoms. Researchers and academics may also find valuable information in studying the underlying causes and potential treatments for this rare disorder.

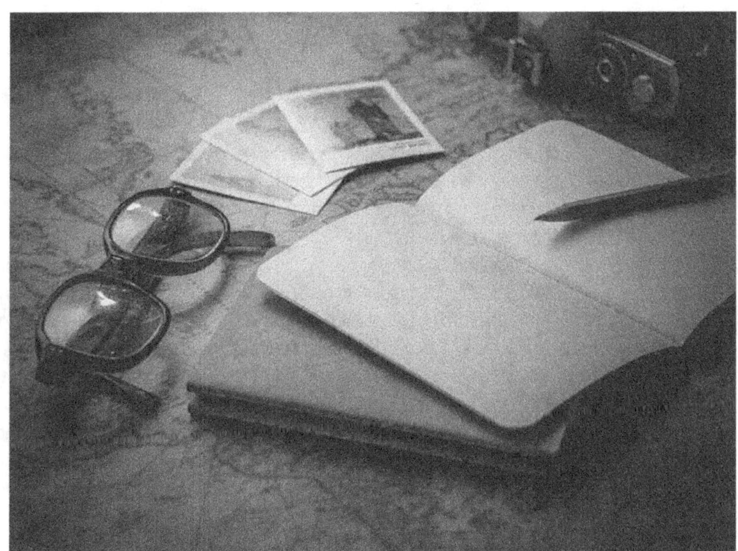

Patients and caregivers affected by Chiari Malformation can find comfort in knowing they are not alone in facing this condition, and may benefit from learning about the experiences of others who have navigated similar challenges. Advocacy groups and NGOs dedicated to supporting individuals with rare brain disorders can also use this information to educate and empower their communities.

Overall, exploring Chiari Malformation sheds light on the complexities of the human brain and the importance of continued research and support for those affected by rare neurological conditions.

Dandy-Walker Syndrome

Dandy-Walker Syndrome is a rare congenital brain malformation that affects the cerebellum, the part of the brain responsible for coordinating movement and balance. This syndrome is characterized by the partial or complete absence of the cerebellar vermis - the structure that connects the two hemispheres of the cerebellum. This anomaly can lead to a variety of neurological and developmental issues, including problems with coordination, muscle tone, and cognitive function.

Individuals with Dandy-Walker Syndrome may exhibit symptoms such as problems with balance and coordination, muscle stiffness or weakness, developmental delays, and intellectual disabilities. In some cases, individuals may also experience hydrocephalus, a condition in which there is an abnormal accumulation of cerebrospinal fluid in the brain, leading to increased pressure inside the skull.

Diagnosing Dandy-Walker Syndrome typically involves a combination of imaging tests, such as MRI or CT scans, to visualize the brain structures and identify any abnormalities. Treatment for this condition often focuses on managing symptoms and complications, such as physical therapy to improve motor skills, medications to control seizures or manage hydrocephalus, and in some cases, surgical intervention to relieve pressure on the brain.

For medical professionals and students, understanding Dandy-Walker Syndrome is crucial for accurately diagnosing and managing patients with this rare condition. By delving into the intricacies of this disorder, healthcare providers can better support individuals with Dandy-Walker Syndrome and their families, offering them the necessary care and resources to improve their quality of life.

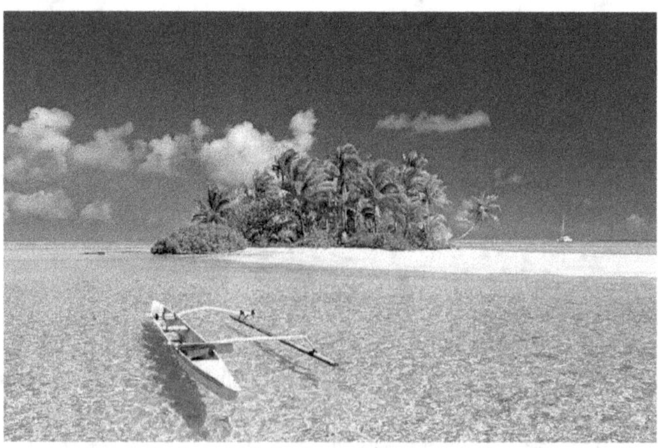

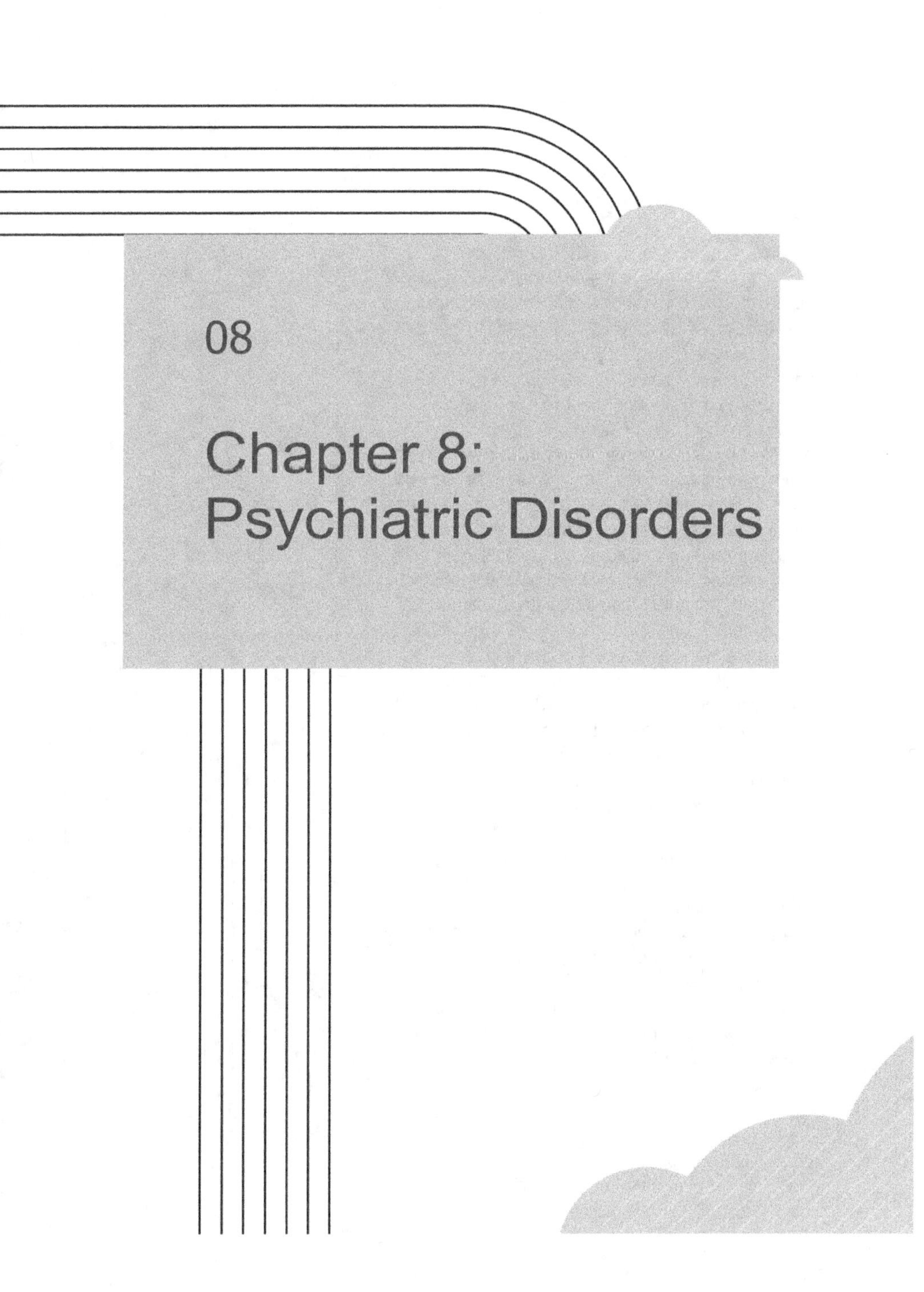

08

Chapter 8:
Psychiatric Disorders

Cotard's Syndrome

Cotard's Syndrome is a rare and perplexing neurological disorder that falls under the category of delusional misidentification syndromes. Also known as Walking Corpse Syndrome, patients with Cotard's Syndrome believe that they are dead, do not exist, or have lost their organs. This delusion can range from a mild feeling of disembodiment to a complete conviction that they are no longer alive.

Medical professionals and students in the fields of neurology and psychiatry may encounter patients with Cotard's Syndrome and must be aware of the unique challenges in diagnosing and treating this disorder. General physicians and nurses may also benefit from understanding the symptoms and potential treatment options for patients presenting with these unusual delusions.

Researchers and academics in the field of neuroscience or psychology can explore the underlying mechanisms of Cotard's Syndrome and contribute to the growing body of knowledge surrounding this mysterious disorder. Medical libraries and institutions may find this chapter on Cotard's Syndrome to be a valuable resource for students and researchers seeking to expand their understanding of less-common neurological conditions.

Patients, caregivers, and advocacy groups dedicated to supporting individuals with rare brain disorders may find comfort in knowing that they are not alone in their struggles with Cotard's Syndrome. By sharing personal stories and insights from medical professionals, this chapter can provide valuable information and support for those affected by this challenging condition.

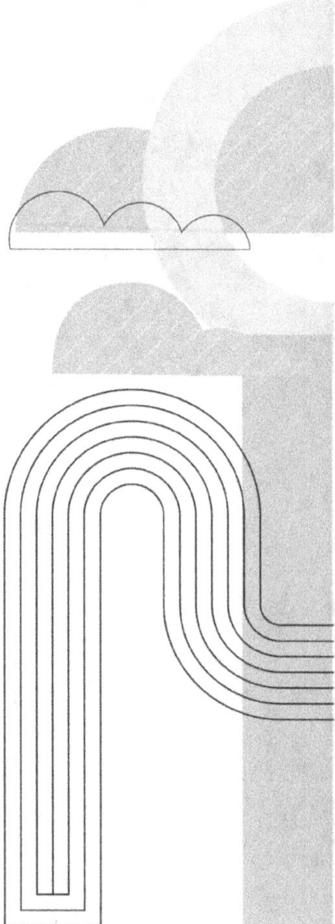

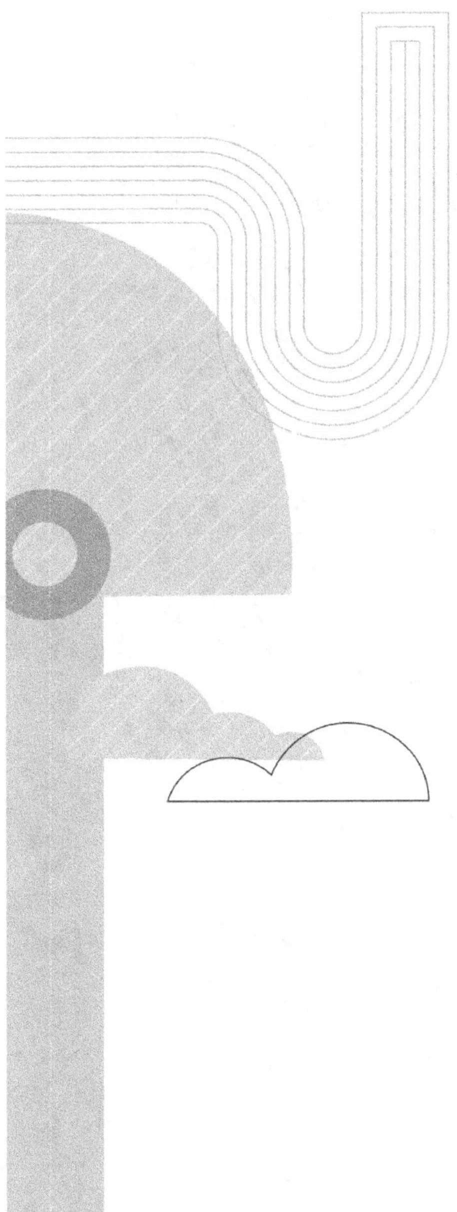

Health enthusiasts, lifelong learners, and non-specialists with a curiosity for the complexities of the human mind may find the exploration of Cotard's Syndrome to be both fascinating and enlightening. By delving into the depths of this mysterious disorder, readers can gain a deeper appreciation for the intricacies of the brain and the diverse range of conditions that can affect its functioning.

Capgras Syndrome

Capgras Syndrome is a rare and fascinating neurological disorder that falls under the umbrella of delusional misidentification syndromes. Patients with Capgras Syndrome firmly believe that a loved one, typically a family member or close friend, has been replaced by an imposter who looks identical to the original person. Despite physical similarities, the individual with Capgras Syndrome is unable to recognize the imposter as the genuine article. The exact cause of Capgras Syndrome remains unknown, but it is believed to stem from a disconnect between the visual processing areas of the brain and the emotional centers responsible for recognizing familiar faces. This disconnection leads to a profound sense of familiarity without the corresponding emotional response, resulting in the delusion of imposters.

Diagnosing Capgras Syndrome can be challenging, as patients often present with a convincing narrative and may not be aware of the irrationality of their beliefs. Treatment typically involves a combination of antipsychotic medication, psychotherapy, and cognitive-behavioral interventions to help patients manage their delusions and improve their quality of life.

Understanding Capgras Syndrome is crucial for medical professionals across various disciplines, as it sheds light on the intricate workings of the human brain and the complex interplay between perception, cognition, and emotion. By delving into the depths of this mysterious disorder, we can gain valuable insights into the inner workings of the mind and develop more effective strategies for diagnosing and treating similar conditions in the future.

Foreign Accent Syndrome

Foreign Accent Syndrome (FAS) is a rare and intriguing neurological disorder that can leave both patients and healthcare professionals baffled. In this subchapter of "Into the Depths of the Mind: Exploring Mysterious Brain Disorders," we delve into the fascinating world of FAS and its impact on individuals.

For medical professionals and students, understanding FAS is crucial in recognizing and diagnosing this rare condition. Neurologists, psychiatrists, general physicians, nurses, and medical students can benefit from learning about the symptoms, causes, and treatment options for patients with FAS. By expanding their knowledge of less-common neurological disorders like FAS, healthcare professionals can better serve their patients and provide appropriate care.

Academics, researchers, and medical librarians may find the information on FAS valuable for academic and research purposes. This subchapter offers insights into the complexities of FAS, shedding light on the underlying mechanisms of this mysterious disorder. By studying FAS, researchers can contribute to the understanding of brain function and language processing.

Patients, caregivers, advocacy groups, and NGOs dedicated to supporting individuals with rare brain disorders can find solace in the detailed information and personal stories shared in this subchapter. By reading about real-life experiences of individuals with FAS, patients and caregivers can gain insights and find support in navigating their journey with this unique condition.

For health enthusiasts, lifelong learners, and non-specialists interested in exploring deep and complex topics related to the human body and its mysteries, the subchapter on FAS offers a window into the enigmatic world of rare brain disorders. By delving into the intricacies of FAS, readers can broaden their understanding of the brain and its remarkable capabilities.

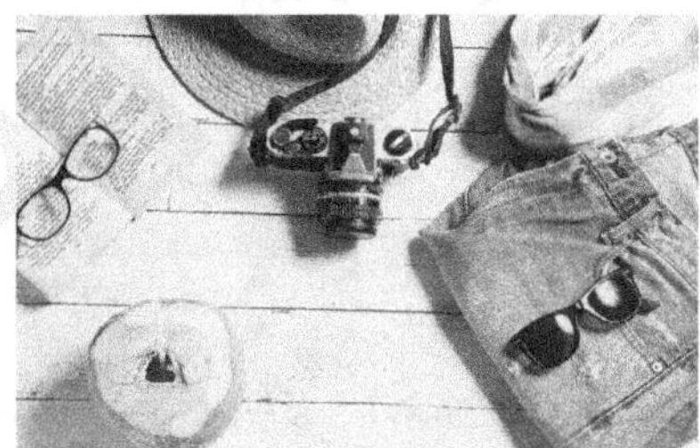

Chapter 9: Conclusion and Future Directions

Challenges in Diagnosing and Treating Rare Brain Disorders

Diagnosing and treating rare brain disorders present unique challenges for medical professionals. Due to their uncommon nature, these disorders often go undiagnosed or misdiagnosed, leading to delays in appropriate treatment. The lack of awareness and limited resources dedicated to researching these conditions further complicates the process.

One of the main challenges in diagnosing rare brain disorders is the variability of symptoms. Patients may present with a wide range of symptoms that overlap with more common neurological conditions, making it difficult for healthcare professionals to pinpoint the exact cause of their illness. Additionally, the lack of standardized diagnostic criteria for many rare disorders adds to the complexity of the diagnostic process.

Treatment of rare brain disorders is also challenging due to the limited understanding of these conditions. Many rare disorders have no known cure, and treatment options are often limited to managing symptoms and improving quality of life. The rarity of these conditions means that there is a lack of research and clinical trials to evaluate the effectiveness of different treatments, leaving healthcare professionals with few evidence-based options.

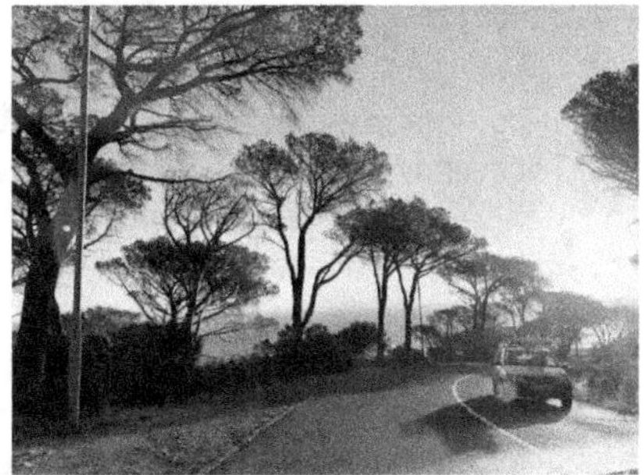

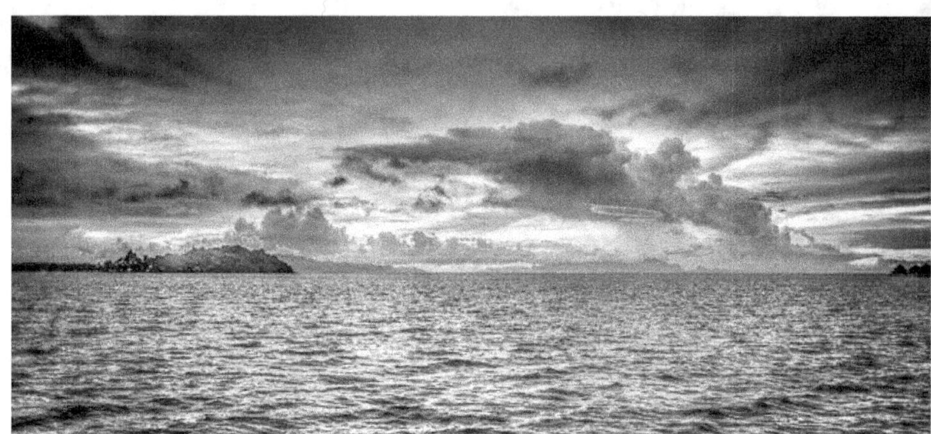

Despite these challenges, advancements in technology and research are providing new insights into rare brain disorders. Collaborations between healthcare professionals, researchers, and advocacy groups are helping to raise awareness and improve diagnosis and treatment options for patients with these conditions.
As we delve into the depths of the mind and explore the mysteries of rare brain disorders, it is essential for medical professionals and researchers to work together to overcome the challenges and provide better care for patients in need. Through continued education, research, and collaboration, we can strive towards improving the diagnosis and treatment of these complex conditions.

The Importance of Research and Advocacy

"The Importance of Research and Advocacy" sheds light on the critical roles that research and advocacy play in understanding and addressing rare and mysterious brain disorders. For medical professionals and students, such as neurologists, psychiatrists, general physicians, nurses, and medical students, this subchapter emphasizes the significance of staying updated on the latest findings and advancements in the field. By engaging in research, medical professionals can contribute to the collective knowledge and potentially discover new treatments or interventions for these less-common neurological conditions.

Academics and researchers, particularly those in neuroscience, psychology, or neurological research, can benefit from the wealth of information provided in this book. The exploration of rare diseases offers a unique opportunity for further study and analysis, potentially leading to breakthroughs in the understanding and management of these complex disorders.

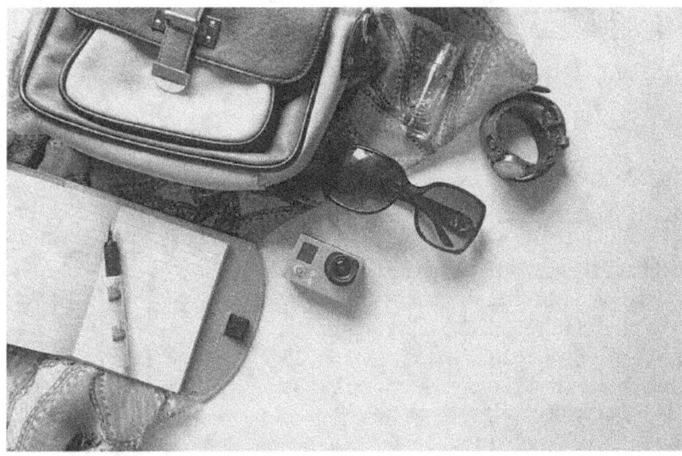

For patients, caregivers, advocacy groups, and NGOs dedicated to supporting individuals with rare brain disorders, this subchapter underscores the importance of raising awareness and advocating for improved resources and support systems. By sharing personal stories and insights, individuals affected by these conditions can find comfort and solidarity in knowing that they are not alone in their journey. Health enthusiasts, lifelong learners, and non-specialists are invited to delve into the depths of the mind through this book, offering a fascinating look into the mysteries of the human brain and the conditions that challenge our understanding. By fostering curiosity and expanding knowledge in this area, readers can gain a deeper appreciation for the complexities of the brain and the importance of ongoing research and advocacy efforts in the field of neurology."

Looking Towards the Future of Understanding and Managing Brain Disorders

As we look towards the future of understanding and managing brain disorders, it is essential for medical professionals and researchers to continue expanding their knowledge and exploring the depths of the mind. "Into the Depths of the Mind: Exploring Mysterious Brain Disorders" offers a comprehensive look at 25 rare and mysterious brain disorders, providing valuable insights and information for a wide range of audiences.

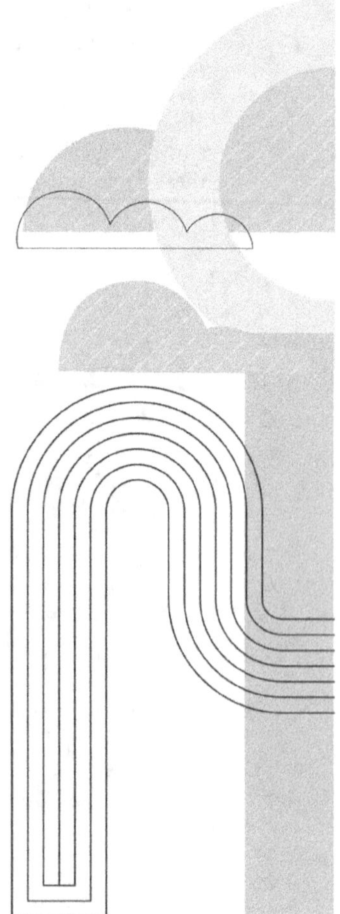

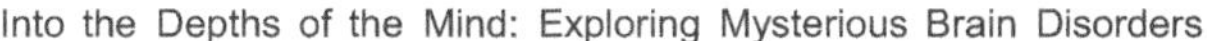

For medical professionals and students, this book serves as a reference guide to broaden their understanding of less-common neurological disorders. Neurologists, psychiatrists, general physicians, nurses, and medical students can benefit from the detailed information and case studies presented in the book.

Academics and researchers involved in neuroscience, psychology, or neurological research will find the collection of rare diseases useful for academic and research purposes. The book offers a unique perspective on lesser-known brain disorders, sparking new ideas and avenues for further study.

Patients, caregivers, advocacy groups, and NGOs dedicated to supporting individuals with rare brain disorders can also find valuable information and personal stories in this book. It serves as an educational resource to inform their work and provide insights and support to those affected by these conditions.

Health enthusiasts, lifelong learners, and non-specialists with a curiosity for the mysteries of the human body will also find "Into the Depths of the Mind" to be a fascinating read. Delving into the complexities of the brain and its disorders, this book offers a captivating journey into the unknown realms of the mind.

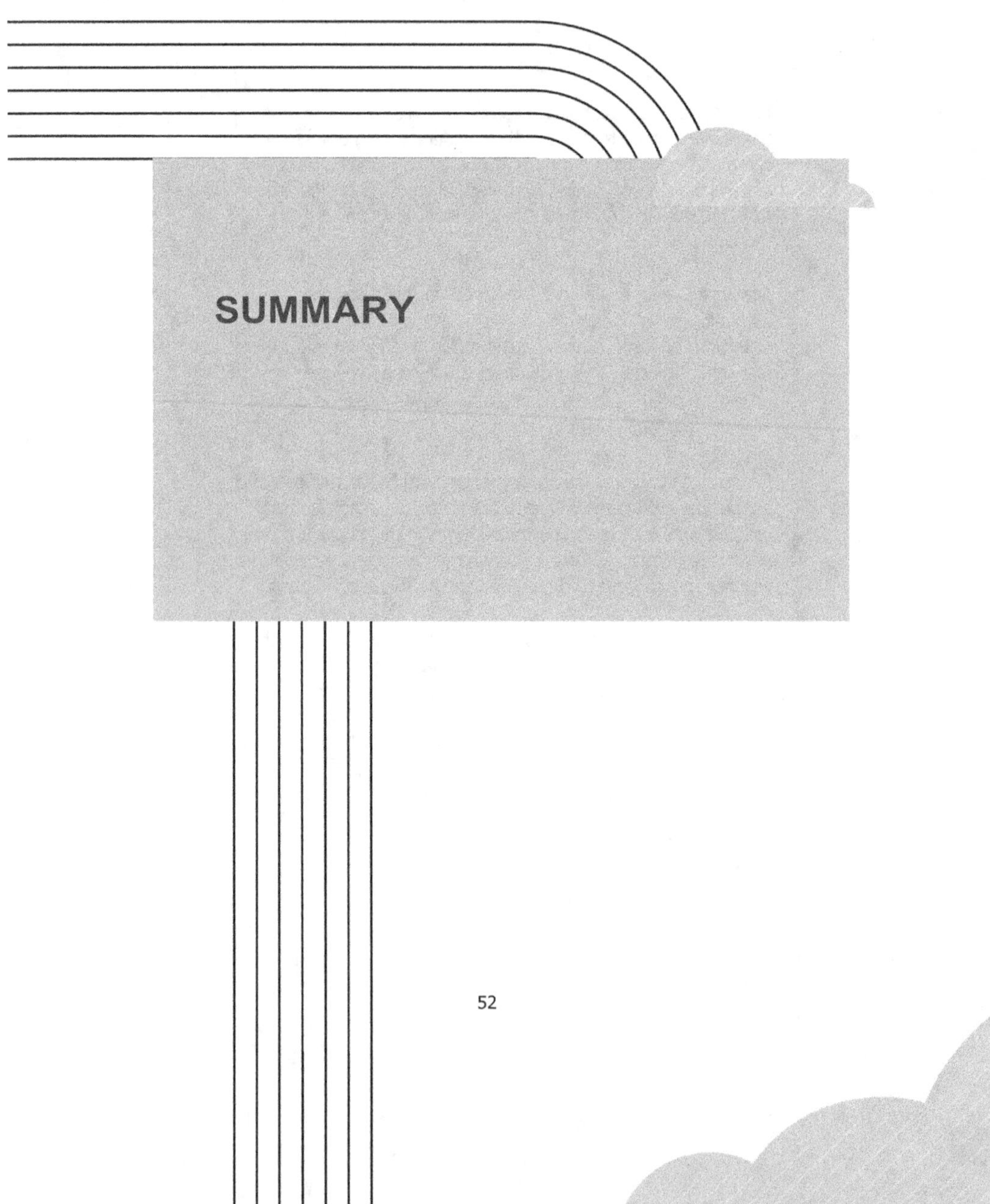
SUMMARY

Creutzfeldt-Jakob Disease

Creutzfeldt-Jakob Disease (CJD) is a rare and fatal degenerative brain disorder that belongs to a group of conditions known as prion diseases. It is characterized by the abnormal folding of proteins in the brain, leading to rapid neurological deterioration.

Definition:
Creutzfeldt-Jakob Disease is a progressive and incurable condition that affects the brain, causing severe cognitive and physical decline. It is believed to be caused by the presence of misfolded prion proteins, which trigger the abnormal folding of normal proteins in the brain.

Symptoms:
Symptoms of CJD typically include rapidly progressing dementia, involuntary muscle movements, difficulty walking, and behavioral changes. As the disease advances, individuals may also experience visual disturbances, hallucinations, and muscle stiffness.

Diagnosis:
Diagnosis of Creutzfeldt-Jakob Disease often involves a combination of clinical evaluation, imaging studies such as MRI or CT scans, cerebrospinal fluid analysis, and sometimes brain biopsies. Additionally, specific electroencephalogram (EEG) patterns can aid in confirming the diagnosis.

Treatment and Survival:
Unfortunately, there is no cure for Creutzfeldt-Jakob Disease, and treatment aims to alleviate symptoms and provide supportive care. The average survival time from diagnosis is typically less than a year, with most individuals succumbing to the disease within a few months of symptom onset. Palliative care and symptom management play a crucial role in enhancing the quality of life for patients with CJD.

Huntington's Disease

Huntington's Disease is a hereditary neurodegenerative disorder that results in the progressive breakdown of nerve cells in the brain. It is characterized by a combination of movement, cognitive, and psychiatric symptoms, with onset typically occurring in adulthood.

Definition:
Huntington's Disease is a genetic condition caused by a mutation in the Huntingtin gene, leading to the production of a faulty protein that damages nerve cells in the brain. The disease is inherited in an autosomal dominant pattern, meaning that a child of an affected individual has a 50% chance of inheriting the mutated gene.

Symptoms:
Symptoms of Huntington's Disease include involuntary movements (chorea), impaired coordination, cognitive decline, psychiatric disturbances such as depression and irritability, and eventually, the loss of the ability to walk, talk, and swallow. The severity and progression of symptoms can vary widely among individuals.

Diagnosis:
Diagnosing Huntington's Disease involves a comprehensive medical history, genetic testing to identify the presence of the mutation, neurological examinations, and imaging tests such as MRI or CT scans to assess brain changes associated with the disease.

Treatment and Survival:
While there is currently no cure for Huntington's Disease, treatment focuses on managing symptoms and improving quality of life. Medications can help alleviate movement disorders and psychiatric symptoms, while therapy and support services can assist with coping strategies. The course of the disease varies, but individuals with Huntington's Disease typically survive for 15-20 years after symptom onset, with care tailored to their evolving needs as the condition progresses.

Progressive Supranuclear Palsy

Progressive Supranuclear Palsy (PSP) is a rare neurodegenerative disorder that affects movement, balance, and cognition. It is characterized by the deterioration of certain brain cells in areas responsible for controlling eye movements and coordination, leading to a range of symptoms that worsen over time.

Definition:
PSP is a progressive brain disorder that results in the accumulation of abnormal tau protein in brain cells, causing impaired control of eye movements, balance difficulties, muscle stiffness, and cognitive changes. It is often misdiagnosed initially due to its resemblance to other neurological conditions like Parkinson's disease.

Symptoms:
Symptoms of PSP include blurred vision, difficulties with eye movements, slowed walking, frequent falls, muscle stiffness, slurred speech, and cognitive impairment. Individuals with PSP may also experience emotional and behavioral changes, such as apathy or irritability.

Diagnosis:
Diagnosing PSP typically involves a thorough neurological examination, medical history review, and imaging tests like MRI or CT scans to evaluate brain structure. Certain eye movement abnormalities, such as the inability to look downward voluntarily, are key diagnostic features. Additionally, cerebrospinal fluid analysis or neuropsychological testing may be conducted to confirm the diagnosis.

Treatment and Survival:
There is currently no cure for PSP, and treatment focuses on managing symptoms to improve quality of life. Medications may help alleviate movement issues, speech therapy can aid communication difficulties, and adaptive devices can enhance mobility. The progression of PSP varies among individuals, but the average survival time after diagnosis ranges from 5 to 10 years, with care often involving a multidisciplinary approach to address the complex needs of individuals with the disease.

Rett Syndrome

Rett Syndrome is a rare genetic neurological disorder that primarily affects girls. It is characterized by a wide range of symptoms that typically emerge in early childhood and lead to severe physical and cognitive impairments.

Definition:
Rett Syndrome is a genetic disorder caused by mutations in the MECP2 gene, which plays a crucial role in brain development. It predominantly affects girls due to its X-linked inheritance pattern. The condition leads to developmental regression, loss of purposeful hand skills, and impaired communication abilities.

Symptoms:
Symptoms of Rett Syndrome include developmental delays, repetitive hand movements (such as wringing or clapping), breathing abnormalities, seizures, apraxia (difficulty with coordinated movements), and social withdrawal. Individuals with Rett Syndrome may also experience cognitive impairments and behavioral challenges.

Diagnosis:
Diagnosing Rett Syndrome involves a thorough clinical evaluation, genetic testing to identify mutations in the MECP2 gene, and assessment of developmental regression and characteristic symptoms. Physical and neurological examinations, as well as developmental assessments, play a crucial role in confirming the diagnosis.

Treatment and Survival:
While there is no cure for Rett Syndrome, treatment aims to manage symptoms and improve quality of life. Therapies such as physical, occupational, and speech therapy can help enhance motor skills and communication abilities. Supportive care, assistive devices, and educational interventions are essential components of treatment. The lifespan of individuals with Rett Syndrome varies, with many living into adulthood, requiring ongoing care and support tailored to their specific needs.

Angelman Syndrome

Angelman Syndrome is a rare genetic disorder that primarily affects the nervous system, leading to severe developmental delays, intellectual disabilities, and unique behavioral characteristics. It is characterized by a distinct neurodevelopmental profile and often presents with a happy demeanor and frequent laughter.

Definition:
Angelman Syndrome is caused by a deletion or mutation in the UBE3A gene, leading to the absence or dysfunction of the UBE3A protein in the brain. This results in developmental delays, speech impairment, movement and balance issues, and a distinctive behavioral phenotype marked by hyperactivity and frequent smiling.

Symptoms:
Symptoms of Angelman Syndrome include developmental delays, speech impairment (often leading to minimal or absent speech), seizures, movement and coordination problems, sleep disturbances, and a happy, excitable demeanor with frequent laughter. Individuals with Angelman Syndrome may also exhibit specific hand movements, such as hand-flapping.

Diagnosis:
Diagnosing Angelman Syndrome involves genetic testing to identify abnormalities in the UBE3A gene, along with clinical evaluation of developmental delays, neurological symptoms, and behavioral characteristics. Additionally, diagnostic criteria include specialized testing for seizures and specific EEG patterns associated with the syndrome.

Treatment and Survival:
While there is no cure for Angelman Syndrome, treatment focuses on managing symptoms and supporting developmental needs. Early intervention services, speech therapy, physical therapy, and behavioral interventions play a crucial role in optimizing outcomes. Seizures are typically managed with anti-epileptic medications. With appropriate care and support, individuals with Angelman Syndrome can lead fulfilling lives. The average lifespan of individuals with Angelman Syndrome aligns with that of the general population, and close monitoring and comprehensive care contribute to improved quality of life.

Fragile X Syndrome

Fragile X Syndrome is a genetic disorder that results in intellectual disabilities, behavioral challenges, and various physical characteristics. It is caused by a mutation in the FMR1 gene, leading to a deficiency of the fragile X mental retardation protein (FMRP) crucial for brain development.

Definition:
Fragile X Syndrome is a genetic condition characterized by a CGG repeat expansion in the FMR1 gene located on the X chromosome. This mutation interferes with the production of FMRP, causing intellectual disabilities, social and communication deficits, hyperactivity, and distinctive physical features such as a long face and large ears.

Symptoms:
Symptoms of Fragile X Syndrome typically include intellectual disabilities, speech and language delays, social anxiety, attention deficits, hyperactivity, sensory sensitivities, and repetitive behaviors. Behavioral challenges, such as impulsivity and aggressive outbursts, are also common among individuals with Fragile X Syndrome.

Diagnosis:
Diagnosing Fragile X Syndrome involves genetic testing to detect the CGG repeat expansion in the FMR1 gene. Clinical evaluation of developmental delays, cognitive functioning, speech and language abilities, and behavioral patterns helps confirm the diagnosis. Family history and physical characteristics may also provide diagnostic clues.

Treatment and Survival:
Management of Fragile X Syndrome focuses on addressing symptoms and providing supportive care. Interventions may include special education programs, speech and occupational therapies, behavioral therapies, and medications to manage symptoms such as anxiety and hyperactivity. While there is no cure for Fragile X Syndrome, early intervention and comprehensive care can significantly improve outcomes and quality of life for individuals with the condition. With appropriate support, many individuals with Fragile X Syndrome live into adulthood, requiring ongoing monitoring and tailored interventions to address their unique needs.

Anti-NMDA Rceptor Encephalitis

Anti-NMDA Receptor Encephalitis is a rare autoimmune disorder that affects the brain, leading to a variety of neurological symptoms and psychiatric manifestations. It is characterized by the body's immune system attacking NMDA receptors in the brain, causing inflammation and dysfunction in the central nervous system.

Definition:
Anti-NMDA Receptor Encephalitis is an autoimmune condition where antibodies target and attack NMDA receptors, which play a crucial role in brain function. This results in inflammation in the brain, leading to symptoms ranging from memory deficits, seizures, and movement disorders to psychiatric symptoms like hallucinations and mood disturbances.

Symptoms:
Symptoms of Anti-NMDA Receptor Encephalitis include cognitive deficits, memory problems, speech and language disturbances, seizures, abnormal movements, hallucinations, psychosis, and behavioral changes. The condition often progresses in stages, with symptoms evolving over time.

Diagnosis:
Diagnosing Anti-NMDA Receptor Encephalitis involves a combination of clinical evaluation, imaging studies such as MRI or CT scans to assess brain inflammation, cerebrospinal fluid analysis for the presence of antibodies, and EEG to monitor brain activity. Testing for NMDA receptor antibodies in the blood or cerebrospinal fluid is crucial for confirming the diagnosis.

Treatment and Survival:
Treatment for Anti-NMDA Receptor Encephalitis typically involves immunotherapy to suppress the immune response and reduce inflammation in the brain. Intravenous immunoglobulin (IVIG), corticosteroids, plasma exchange, and in severe cases, rituximab or cyclophosphamide may be used. Early diagnosis and prompt treatment are essential for a better outcome, as delays in care can increase the risk of long-term neurological complications. Survival rates vary, with timely and aggressive treatment significantly improving prognosis and quality of life for individuals with the condition.

Stiff Person Syndrome (SPS)

Stiff Person Syndrome is a rare neurological disorder characterized by muscle stiffness and continuous muscle contractions, leading to significant disability and impaired mobility. It affects the central nervous system and primarily affects the muscles of the trunk and limbs.

Definition:
Stiff Person Syndrome is a neurological condition marked by severe muscle stiffness, spasms, and rigidity, often triggered by stress, noise, or sudden movements. The underlying cause of SPS is thought to be an autoimmune response that disrupts the communication between the brain and spinal cord.

Symptoms:
Symptoms of Stiff Person Syndrome include muscle rigidity, exaggerated startle reflex (hyperekplexia), muscle spasms, and stiffness that can lead to postural abnormalities and difficulty moving. Patients may also experience anxiety, fear, and emotional distress triggered by muscle stiffness episodes.

Diagnosis:
Diagnosing Stiff Person Syndrome involves a thorough clinical examination, assessment of symptoms, electromyography (EMG) to measure muscle activity, and blood tests to check for antibodies associated with autoimmune responses. Neurological imaging may also be used to rule out other conditions.

Treatment and Survival:
Treatment for Stiff Person Syndrome aims to manage symptoms and improve quality of life. Medications such as benzodiazepines, muscle relaxants, and immunosuppressants may be prescribed to alleviate muscle stiffness and spasms. Physical therapy, cognitive-behavioral therapy, and counseling can help manage emotional aspects of the condition. Survival in individuals with Stiff Person Syndrome varies, with many individuals experiencing fluctuating symptoms that can be managed with a multidisciplinary approach to care. Early diagnosis and appropriate symptom management are crucial for optimizing outcomes and enhancing quality of life for those living with SPS.

Neuromyelitis Optica

Neuromyelitis Optica (NMO), also known as Devic's Disease, is a rare autoimmune disorder that primarily affects the optic nerve and spinal cord, leading to inflammation and damage of these crucial components of the central nervous system.

Definition:
Neuromyelitis Optica is characterized by recurrent episodes of inflammation in the optic nerve (optic neuritis) and the spinal cord (myelitis). It is caused by the immune system attacking aquaporin-4, a protein found in the central nervous system, leading to neuroinflammation, demyelination, and nerve cell damage.

Symptoms:
Symptoms of Neuromyelitis Optica can include visual disturbances, such as vision loss or blurred vision, weakness or paralysis in the limbs, numbness, sensory disturbances, and bladder and bowel dysfunction. Additionally, individuals with NMO may experience episodes of severe pain and neurological deficits.

Diagnosis:
Diagnosing Neuromyelitis Optica involves a combination of clinical evaluation, imaging studies such as MRI to detect characteristic lesions in the optic nerve and spinal cord, blood tests to check for aquaporin-4 antibodies, and examination of cerebrospinal fluid for signs of inflammation.

Treatment and Survival:
Treatment for Neuromyelitis Optica aims to suppress the immune response, reduce inflammation, and prevent relapses. Immunosuppressive therapies, corticosteroids, plasma exchange, and newer biologic agents are commonly used to manage the symptoms and prevent disease progression. Early diagnosis and prompt treatment are crucial for improving outcomes and quality of life for individuals with NMO, as aggressive management can help prevent disability and improve long-term survival. The outlook for individuals with Neuromyelitis Optica varies, with many individuals experiencing relapsing episodes that can be managed with proper medical care and ongoing monitoring.

Neurocysticercosis

Neurocysticercosis is a parasitic infection of the central nervous system caused by the larval form of the pork tapeworm, Taenia solium. It occurs when the parasite's larvae migrate to the brain or spinal cord, leading to a range of neurological symptoms and potentially severe complications.

Definition:
Neurocysticercosis is a condition resulting from the development of cysts containing the larval stage of Taenia solium in the brain or spinal cord. When these cysts form within the central nervous system, they can lead to inflammation, tissue damage, and a variety of neurological manifestations.

Symptoms:
Symptoms of Neurocysticercosis can vary widely depending on the location and number of cysts present. Common symptoms include headaches, seizures, cognitive impairment, visual disturbances, balance problems, and in severe cases, hydrocephalus or stroke-like symptoms.

Diagnosis:
Diagnosing Neurocysticercosis involves a combination of clinical assessment, imaging studies such as MRI or CT scans to detect cysts in the brain or spinal cord, serological tests to detect antibodies against Taenia solium, and sometimes cerebrospinal fluid analysis to confirm the presence of the parasite.

Treatment and Survival:
Treatment for Neurocysticercosis typically involves a combination of antiparasitic medication to kill the cysticerci, corticosteroids to reduce inflammation, and in some cases, surgical intervention to resect cysts causing mass effect. Prompt and appropriate treatment is essential to prevent complications and improve outcomes. With timely intervention, many individuals with Neurocysticercosis can recover fully or manage their symptoms effectively. However, in severe cases with complications like hydrocephalus or brain damage, the prognosis may be less favorable, emphasizing the importance of early detection and comprehensive care.

Progressive Multifocal Leukoencephalopathy (PML)

PML is a rare and severe viral infection of the brain caused by the JC virus, which leads to the destruction of myelin, the protective covering of nerve cells. PML primarily affects individuals with weakened immune systems, such as those with HIV/AIDS, undergoing immunosuppressive therapy, or with certain autoimmune conditions.

Definition:
Progressive Multifocal Leukoencephalopathy is characterized by the demyelination of nerve cells in multiple areas of the brain, leading to progressive neurological deficits. The JC virus, which typically remains dormant in the body, can become reactivated and cause PML in individuals with compromised immune function.

Symptoms:
Symptoms of Progressive Multifocal Leukoencephalopathy can include weakness, clumsiness, cognitive decline, visual disturbances, difficulty speaking or understanding language, and in severe cases, paralysis. The progression of symptoms tends to be rapid and can lead to significant disability.

Diagnosis:
Diagnosing Progressive Multifocal Leukoencephalopathy involves neurological evaluation, imaging studies such as MRI to detect characteristic lesions in the brain, and sometimes cerebrospinal fluid analysis to confirm the presence of the JC virus. Biopsy may be necessary in some cases to definitively diagnose PML.

Treatment and Survival:
Treatment for Progressive Multifocal Leukoencephalopathy focuses on managing symptoms and controlling the underlying immune deficiency. Antiretroviral therapy for HIV/AIDS, reduction of immunosuppressive medications, and potentially antiviral agents to target the JC virus may be considered. Prognosis and survival vary depending on the immune status of the individual and the extent of neurological damage. Despite advances in treatment, PML remains a challenging condition with a high risk of morbidity and mortality, especially in individuals with severely compromised immune systems. Early detection and intervention are crucial to potentially improve outcomes and quality of life for those affected by PML.

Variant Creutzfeldt-Jakob Disease

Variant Creutzfeldt-Jakob Disease (vCJD) is a rare and fatal prion disease that affects the brain, leading to rapid neurological deterioration and severe cognitive impairment. It is believed to be caused by the consumption of contaminated beef products containing abnormal prion proteins.

Definition:
Variant Creutzfeldt-Jakob Disease is a form of transmissible spongiform encephalopathy caused by abnormal prion proteins, leading to the formation of tiny holes in the brain tissue. The disease primarily affects younger individuals and is linked to exposure to bovine spongiform encephalopathy (mad cow disease).

Symptoms:
Symptoms of Variant Creutzfeldt-Jakob Disease include progressive cognitive decline, memory loss, personality changes, muscle stiffness, coordination problems, visual disturbances, and eventually, a profound state of dementia. Individuals affected by vCJD typically experience rapid deterioration in neurological function.

Diagnosis:
Diagnosing Variant Creutzfeldt-Jakob Disease involves a clinical assessment of symptoms, neurological examinations, imaging studies such as MRI to evaluate brain changes, and potentially EEG to monitor brain activity. Definitive diagnosis often requires brain biopsy or post-mortem examination.

Treatment and Survival:
There is currently no cure for Variant Creutzfeldt-Jakob Disease, and treatment focuses on managing symptoms and providing supportive care. Palliative interventions aimed at improving quality of life and minimizing discomfort are typically provided. The prognosis for vCJD is poor, with rapid progression of symptoms leading to severe disability within a few months to years following diagnosis. Unfortunately, vCJD is ultimately fatal, and survival beyond a few years is uncommon. Extensive supportive care and compassionate end-of-life care are crucial for individuals and families affected by this devastating and untreatable condition.

Wilson's Disease

Wilson's Disease is a rare inherited disorder characterized by the body's inability to properly metabolize copper, leading to the accumulation of excess copper in various tissues, particularly the liver and brain. This build-up of copper can cause severe damage and lead to a variety of symptoms affecting the liver, nervous system, and other organs.

Definition:
Wilson's Disease is caused by mutations in the ATP7B gene, which is responsible for the transport of copper in the body. When this gene is defective, copper cannot be excreted properly, resulting in toxic levels of copper accumulating in the liver, brain, and other tissues.

Symptoms:
Symptoms of Wilson's Disease can vary widely and may include liver problems such as jaundice, hepatitis, and cirrhosis, neurological symptoms like tremors, difficulty speaking or swallowing, psychiatric disturbances, and eye issues such as Kayser-Fleischer rings. The condition can also manifest as behavioral changes or cognitive impairment.

Diagnosis:
Diagnosing Wilson's Disease involves a combination of clinical evaluation, laboratory tests to measure copper levels in the blood and urine, genetic testing to identify mutations in the ATP7B gene, and liver imaging studies to assess liver damage. Other diagnostic tools may include eye exams and neurological assessments.

Treatment and Survival:
Treatment for Wilson's Disease aims to reduce copper levels in the body and prevent further copper accumulation. This typically involves long-term use of medications such as chelating agents or zinc to promote copper excretion. In severe cases, liver transplantation may be necessary to manage liver failure. With appropriate and timely treatment, individuals with Wilson's Disease can lead relatively normal lives. However, early diagnosis and lifelong management are essential for optimizing outcomes and preventing complications such as liver failure or neurological damage. With proper care, many individuals with Wilson's Disease can have a normal lifespan.

Maple Syrup Urine Disease

Maple Syrup Urine Disease (MSUD) is a rare inherited metabolic disorder that interferes with the body's ability to break down certain amino acids, resulting in a buildup of toxic substances in the blood and urine. The condition gets its name from the distinctive sweet, maple syrup-like odor of the urine in affected individuals.

Definition:
Maple Syrup Urine Disease is caused by mutations in genes responsible for the breakdown of the branched-chain amino acids leucine, isoleucine, and valine. This leads to the accumulation of toxic byproducts that can affect brain function and cause neurological damage, if left untreated.

Symptoms:
Symptoms of Maple Syrup Urine Disease can include poor feeding, lethargy, vomiting, seizures, muscle stiffness, developmental delays, and the characteristic sweet-smelling urine. If untreated, MSUD can lead to severe neurological complications, coma, and even death.

Diagnosis:
Diagnosing Maple Syrup Urine Disease involves newborn screening tests that detect elevated levels of amino acids in the blood or urine, genetic testing to identify mutations in the responsible genes, and further metabolic testing to confirm the diagnosis. In some cases, urine analysis may reveal the characteristic sweet odor.

Treatment and Survival:
Treatment for Maple Syrup Urine Disease focuses on managing the dietary intake of protein and amino acids through a specialized low-protein diet, as well as supplementation with special formulas that help maintain metabolic balance. Regular monitoring and medical management are essential to prevent metabolic crises and neurological damage. With early diagnosis and strict adherence to dietary restrictions, individuals with MSUD can lead relatively normal lives. However, without proper treatment, MSUD can lead to severe complications and may be life-threatening. Compliance with dietary therapy and close medical supervision are key factors in ensuring a good prognosis and long-term survival for individuals with Maple Syrup Urine Disease.

Adrenoleukodystrophy

Adrenoleukodystrophy (ALD) is a rare genetic disorder that affects the nervous system, adrenal glands, and other organs. It is characterized by the buildup of very long-chain fatty acids in various tissues, leading to damage to the myelin sheath surrounding nerve cells in the brain and spinal cord.

Definition:
Adrenoleukodystrophy is caused by mutations in the ABCD1 gene, which impairs the function of a protein involved in the breakdown of very long-chain fatty acids. Accumulation of these fatty acids can lead to deterioration of the myelin sheath, affecting nerve signal transmission and causing neurological dysfunction.

Symptoms:
Symptoms of Adrenoleukodystrophy can vary depending on the type and severity of the condition but may include vision loss, difficulty swallowing, speech and motor impairments, adrenal insufficiency, behavioral changes, and cognitive decline. In its most severe form, ALD can progress rapidly and lead to significant disability or even death.

Diagnosis:
Diagnosing Adrenoleukodystrophy involves genetic testing to identify mutations in the ABCD1 gene, blood tests to measure levels of very long-chain fatty acids, imaging studies such as MRI to assess brain abnormalities, and adrenal function tests to evaluate adrenal gland involvement.

Treatment and Survival:
Treatment for Adrenoleukodystrophy focuses on managing symptoms and slowing disease progression. This may include dietary modifications, hormone replacement therapy for adrenal insufficiency, and potentially stem cell transplantation in some cases to halt the progression of cerebral ALD. The prognosis for individuals with ALD varies depending on the type and stage of the disease, with early detection and intervention being crucial for better outcomes. While there is no cure for Adrenoleukodystrophy, supportive care and appropriate medical management can help improve quality of life and potentially extend survival for affected individuals.

Agenesis of the Corpus Callosum

Agenesis of the Corpus Callosum (ACC) is a rare congenital condition characterized by the complete or partial absence of the corpus callosum, the structure that connects the two hemispheres of the brain. This developmental disorder can lead to a range of neurological and cognitive challenges.

Definition:
Agenesis of the Corpus Callosum is a congenital disorder that occurs when the corpus callosum, the bundle of nerve fibers that facilitates communication between the right and left hemispheres of the brain, fails to develop fully or is absent. This can result in various neurological and developmental abnormalities.

Symptoms:
Individuals with Agenesis of the Corpus Callosum may present with a wide spectrum of symptoms, including intellectual disabilities, developmental delays, motor deficits, seizures, sensory processing issues, and social or behavioral challenges. The severity and type of symptoms can vary depending on the extent of the callosal absence.

Diagnosis:
Diagnosing Agenesis of the Corpus Callosum involves neurological examinations, imaging studies such as MRI to visualize the brain structure, and other tests to assess cognitive and motor function. Genetic testing may also be considered to identify associated genetic conditions.

Treatment and Survival:
Treatment for Agenesis of the Corpus Callosum focuses on managing symptoms and providing supportive care to address specific needs, such as physical therapy for motor impairments or speech therapy for communication difficulties. Early intervention services and educational support are important for individuals with ACC to optimize their development and quality of life. The survival and long-term outcomes for individuals with Agenesis of the Corpus Callosum can vary widely, depending on the presence of associated conditions and the severity of neurological impairments. Comprehensive and personalized care can help individuals with ACC thrive and reach their full potential despite the challenges posed by this congenital brain abnormality.

Chiari Malformation

Chiari Malformation is a structural defect in the base of the skull where the cerebellum extends into the spinal canal, compressing the brainstem and disrupting normal cerebrospinal fluid flow. This condition can lead to various neurological symptoms and complications affecting the brain and spinal cord.

Definition:
Chiari Malformation is characterized by the displacement of the cerebellar tonsils through the foramen magnum, the opening at the base of the skull. This can obstruct the flow of cerebrospinal fluid and lead to hydrocephalus or syringomyelia, causing symptoms related to increased pressure in the brain.

Symptoms:
Symptoms of Chiari Malformation can include headaches, neck pain, dizziness, vision problems, balance issues, difficulty swallowing, muscle weakness, and sensory abnormalities. In severe cases, individuals may experience breathing difficulties or paralysis due to compression of the brainstem.

Diagnosis:
Diagnosing Chiari Malformation involves a thorough neurological examination, imaging studies such as MRI to visualize the brain and spinal cord, and assessment of symptoms to determine the presence and severity of cerebellar herniation. Additional tests may be performed to evaluate associated complications.

Treatment and Survival:
Treatment for Chiari Malformation may include surgical interventions to decompress the cerebellum and restore normal fluid circulation. Different surgical techniques can be utilized based on the individual's symptoms and anatomical features. With prompt diagnosis and appropriate management, many individuals with Chiari Malformation can experience improvement in symptoms and quality of life. The prognosis for Chiari Malformation varies depending on the severity of symptoms, the presence of related conditions, and the response to treatment. Early intervention and ongoing monitoring are essential for optimizing outcomes and potentially preventing long-term complications associated with this neurological disorder.

Chiari Malformation

Definition:
Chiari Malformation is a structural abnormality in which the lower part of the cerebellum, known as the cerebellar tonsils, extends into the foramen magnum (the opening at the base of the skull), causing compression and disruption of normal cerebrospinal fluid flow. There are different types of Chiari Malformation, with Type I being the most common and Type II typically associated with a more severe form of the condition.

Symptoms:
Symptoms of Chiari Malformation can vary widely and may include headaches, neck pain, dizziness, balance problems, difficulty swallowing, numbness or tingling in the extremities, tinnitus, vision changes, and in some cases, breathing difficulties. The presentation of symptoms can be influenced by the type and severity of the malformation.

Diagnosis:
Diagnosing Chiari Malformation involves a neurological examination, imaging studies such as MRI or CT scans to visualize the brain and spinal cord, and assessment of symptoms. Additional tests such as a spinal tap (lumbar puncture) may be performed to evaluate cerebrospinal fluid pressure.

Treatment and Survival:
Treatment for Chiari Malformation depends on the severity of symptoms and complications. In mild cases, conservative management with pain control and monitoring may be sufficient. However, in cases where symptoms are significant or progressive, surgical intervention to decompress the affected area may be recommended. With appropriate treatment, many individuals with Chiari Malformation can experience symptom relief and improved quality of life. The prognosis largely depends on the presence of associated conditions, the type and severity of the malformation, and the response to treatment. Early diagnosis and comprehensive care are essential in managing Chiari Malformation and optimizing outcomes for affected individuals.

Dandy-Walker Syndrome

Definition:
Dandy-Walker Syndrome is a rare congenital brain malformation that involves the development of a cystic pouch in the fourth ventricle of the brain, abnormal formation of the cerebellum, and enlargement of the posterior fossa. This condition can lead to a range of neurological and developmental impairments.

Symptoms:
Symptoms of Dandy-Walker Syndrome can include developmental delays, motor deficits, coordination problems, hydrocephalus (accumulation of fluid in the brain), intellectual disabilities, and vision abnormalities. Some individuals may also experience increased intracranial pressure, leading to headaches, nausea, and vomiting.

Diagnosis:
Diagnosing Dandy-Walker Syndrome typically involves neurological examinations, imaging studies such as MRI or CT scans to visualize the brain structure, and assessment of symptoms. Additional tests may be performed to evaluate potential complications such as hydrocephalus.

Treatment and Survival:
Treatment for Dandy-Walker Syndrome aims to manage symptoms, prevent complications, and support developmental progress. This may involve monitoring and addressing fluid build-up in the brain, surgical interventions to relieve pressure, and supportive therapies to address cognitive and motor challenges. The prognosis for individuals with Dandy-Walker Syndrome can vary depending on the severity of symptoms, the presence of associated conditions, and the response to treatment. Early intervention, coordinated care, and ongoing support are crucial for optimizing outcomes and improving the quality of life for individuals affected by this congenital brain malformation.

Cotard's Syndrome

Definition:
Cotard's Syndrome, also known as Cotard Delusion or Walking Corpse Syndrome, is a rare neuropsychiatric condition characterized by the delusional belief that one is dead, does not exist, or has lost vital organs or blood. This syndrome is often associated with severe depression, psychosis, or other mental health disorders.

Symptoms:
Individuals with Cotard's Syndrome may experience a range of symptoms, including nihilistic delusions, feelings of emptiness or non-existence, self-neglect, auditory hallucinations, and a disconnection from reality. Some may also exhibit depressive symptoms, anxiety, and cognitive impairments.

Diagnosis:
Diagnosing Cotard's Syndrome involves a comprehensive psychiatric evaluation, including a detailed assessment of the individual's symptoms, medical history, and mental status. Psychological testing, neuroimaging studies, and laboratory tests may be used to rule out other potential causes of the delusional beliefs.

Treatment and Survival:
Treatment for Cotard's Syndrome typically involves a combination of psychotherapy, medication, and supportive care. Cognitive-behavioral therapy, antidepressants, antipsychotic medications, and mood stabilizers may be used to manage delusions, improve mood, and address underlying mental health issues. The prognosis for individuals with Cotard's Syndrome can vary depending on the severity of symptoms, the presence of comorbid conditions, and the response to treatment. With appropriate care and support, many individuals with this rare condition can achieve symptom relief and improve their quality of life. Early intervention and ongoing management are essential in addressing the complex mental health challenges associated with Cotard's Syndrome.

Capgras Syndrome

Definition:
Capgras Syndrome, also known as Capgras Delusion, is a rare psychiatric disorder characterized by the delusional belief that a familiar person, typically a family member, has been replaced by an identical impostor. This condition is often associated with underlying psychiatric conditions such as schizophrenia, dementia, or brain injury.

Symptoms:
Individuals with Capgras Syndrome may exhibit the delusional belief that someone close to them has been replaced by an identical imposter, despite the person's physical resemblance and behavior. Other symptoms may include paranoia, anxiety, confusion, and emotional detachment from the supposed impostor.

Diagnosis:
Diagnosing Capgras Syndrome involves a thorough psychiatric evaluation, including a detailed assessment of the individual's symptoms, medical history, and mental status. Psychological testing, neuroimaging studies, and laboratory tests may be used to rule out other potential causes of delusional beliefs.

Treatment and Survival:
Treatment for Capgras Syndrome typically involves a combination of psychotherapy, medication, and supportive care. Cognitive-behavioral therapy, antipsychotic medications, and mood stabilizers may be used to address delusions, manage underlying psychological issues, and improve overall mental health. The prognosis for individuals with Capgras Syndrome depends on the severity of symptoms, the presence of comorbid conditions, and the individual's response to treatment. With appropriate care and support, many individuals with this rare condition can experience symptom relief and improved quality of life. Early intervention and ongoing management are essential in addressing the complex psychiatric challenges associated with Capgras Syndrome.

Foreign Accent Syndrome

Definition:
Foreign Accent Syndrome is a rare speech disorder characterized by the sudden onset of speech changes that make an individual's accent sound foreign to their native language, even though they have not acquired a new accent. This condition may result from neurological conditions, such as stroke, brain injury, or other underlying neurological disorders.

Symptoms:
Individuals with Foreign Accent Syndrome may present with altered speech patterns, intonation, and articulation that resemble a foreign accent, even though the language being spoken remains the same. The perceived accent change can lead to communication difficulties, social challenges, and emotional distress for those affected by the condition.

Diagnosis:
Diagnosing Foreign Accent Syndrome involves a comprehensive neurological evaluation, including a detailed assessment of the individual's speech patterns, medical history, and neurological symptoms. Imaging studies, such as MRI or CT scans, may be used to identify underlying brain abnormalities or damage that could be contributing to the speech changes.

Treatment and Survival:
Treatment for Foreign Accent Syndrome focuses on speech therapy and rehabilitation to help individuals improve their communication skills, articulate speech more clearly, and adapt to the changes in their accent. The prognosis for individuals with Foreign Accent Syndrome largely depends on the underlying cause of the condition, the severity of speech changes, and the individual's response to therapy. With proper intervention and support, many individuals with this rare speech disorder can learn to manage their symptoms and improve their ability to communicate effectively. Early diagnosis and tailored treatment plans are essential in helping individuals overcome the challenges associated with Foreign Accent Syndrome.

Moyamoya Disease

Definition:
Moyamoya Disease is a rare cerebrovascular disorder characterized by the progressive narrowing or blockage of the internal carotid arteries in the brain, leading to the formation of tiny blood vessels to compensate for reduced blood flow. The term "moyamoya" means "puff of smoke" in Japanese, describing the appearance of the fragile, interconnected blood vessels that develop in response to the arterial blockages.

Symptoms:
Symptoms of Moyamoya Disease can vary but often include recurrent strokes, transient ischemic attacks (mini-strokes), headaches, seizures, cognitive impairments, and weakness or paralysis in limbs. Children may present with developmental delays and deficits in learning and behavior.

Diagnosis:
Diagnosing Moyamoya Disease typically involves imaging studies such as MRI, CT angiography, or cerebral angiography to visualize the narrowed blood vessels and collateral vessel formation characteristic of the condition. Neurological evaluations and cognitive assessments may also be performed to assess the extent of brain involvement.

Treatment and Survival:
Treatment for Moyamoya Disease aims to improve blood flow to the brain and prevent further strokes. Surgical interventions such as direct or indirect revascularization procedures may be recommended to create new pathways for blood flow. Medications to manage risk factors for stroke, such as high blood pressure and clotting disorders, may also be prescribed. The prognosis for individuals with Moyamoya Disease largely depends on the severity of symptoms, the progression of the disease, and the response to treatment. With appropriate care and management, many individuals with Moyamoya Disease can experience improved quality of life and reduced risk of complications associated with decreased blood flow to the brain. Early diagnosis and intervention are crucial in optimizing outcomes for individuals affected by this rare cerebrovascular disorder.

Sydenham's Chorea (St. Vitus Dance)

Definition:
Sydenham's Chorea, also known as St. Vitus Dance, is a rare neurological disorder that primarily affects children and adolescents. It is characterized by the development of involuntary, rapid, jerky movements of the face, arms, and legs, along with muscle weakness, emotional disturbances, and sometimes cognitive impairments. Sydenham's Chorea is often associated with rheumatic fever, an inflammatory condition that can result from untreated streptococcal infections.

Symptoms:
Symptoms of Sydenham's Chorea include choreiform movements (sudden, purposeless movements), muscle weakness, impaired coordination, emotional lability, and behavioral changes. Children may also experience difficulties with fine motor skills, walking, and balance, impacting their daily functioning and quality of life.

Diagnosis:
Diagnosing Sydenham's Chorea typically involves a thorough medical history, physical examination, and neurological assessments to evaluate the characteristic movement abnormalities and associated symptoms. Laboratory tests may be conducted to assess for markers of inflammation and evidence of recent streptococcal infection.

Treatment and Survival:
Treatment for Sydenham's Chorea focuses on managing symptoms and addressing the underlying cause, often through the use of medications to reduce inflammation, control movement disorders, and treat streptococcal infections. Physical therapy and psychotherapy may also be recommended to help improve motor skills, emotional regulation, and quality of life. With prompt treatment and appropriate management, many individuals with Sydenham's Chorea can experience symptom relief and significant improvement in motor function and cognitive abilities. The prognosis for individuals with Sydenham's Chorea is generally favorable, with most cases resolving over time, especially if treated promptly and effectively. Early diagnosis and multidisciplinary care are essential in optimizing outcomes for individuals affected by this rare neurological disorder.

Balo's Concentric Sclerosis

Definition:
Balo's Concentric Sclerosis is a rare demyelinating disorder of the central nervous system characterized by the formation of concentric rings of demyelination within the brain. This distinct pattern of demyelination gives the lesions a target-like appearance when visualized on imaging studies. The cause of Balo's Concentric Sclerosis is not fully understood, but it is believed to involve autoimmune mechanisms attacking the myelin sheath.

Symptoms:
Symptoms of Balo's Concentric Sclerosis can vary but often include neurological deficits such as weakness, visual disturbances, coordination problems, cognitive impairments, and sensory abnormalities. The presentation may be acute or subacute, with symptoms worsening over time.

Diagnosis:
Diagnosing Balo's Concentric Sclerosis involves brain imaging studies such as MRI or CT scans to visualize the characteristic concentric rings of demyelination. A lumbar puncture may be performed to analyze cerebrospinal fluid for markers of inflammation. Biopsy of brain tissue may also be necessary for definitive diagnosis.

Treatment and Survival:
Treatment for Balo's Concentric Sclerosis focuses on managing symptoms and slowing disease progression. High-dose steroids, immunosuppressive medications, and plasma exchange therapy may be used to reduce inflammation and modulate the immune response. Physical therapy and supportive care can help manage symptoms and improve quality of life. The prognosis for individuals with Balo's Concentric Sclerosis varies depending on the extent of demyelination and the response to treatment. Some individuals may experience periods of remission, while others may have a more progressive course. Early diagnosis and multidisciplinary care are crucial in optimizing outcomes for individuals affected by this rare demyelinating disorder.

10

Appendix: Resources for Further Reading and Support

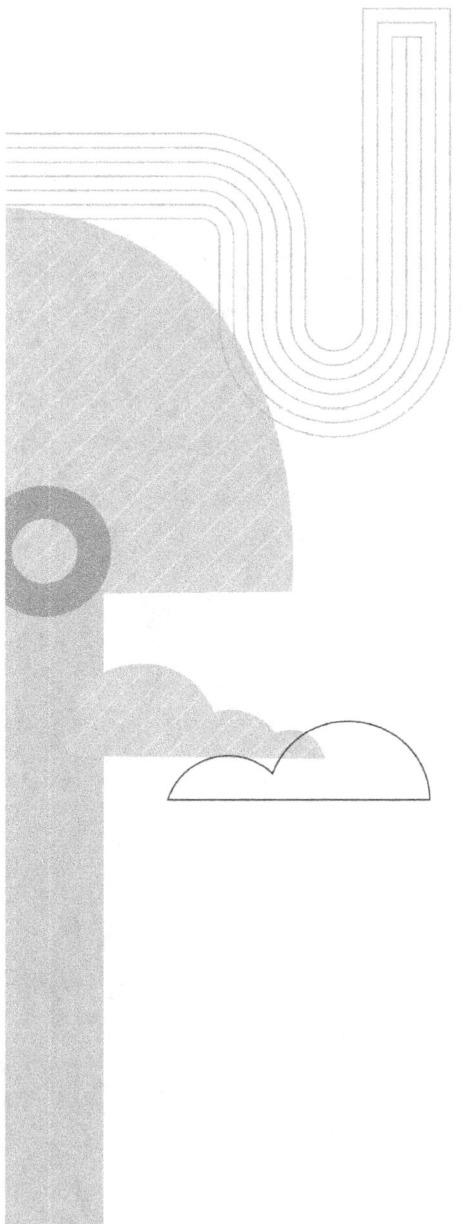

In the appendix of "Into the Depths of the Mind: Exploring Mysterious Brain Disorders," readers will find a curated list of resources for further reading and support related to the rare and mysterious brain disorders discussed in the book. This section is designed to provide medical professionals, researchers, patients, caregivers, advocacy groups, and other interested individuals with additional information and tools to deepen their understanding of these complex conditions.

For medical professionals and students, the appendix includes references to specialized medical journals, academic papers, and professional organizations that focus on neurology, psychiatry, and rare neurological disorders. These resources can serve as valuable sources of information for those looking to expand their knowledge and expertise in this area.

Academics and researchers will also find the appendix to be a valuable resource, as it includes references to research studies, clinical trials, and academic conferences related to the rare brain disorders discussed in the book. These resources can help researchers stay up to date on the latest developments in the field and connect with other experts in the field.

Patients, caregivers, and advocacy groups can benefit from the appendix by finding support groups, patient organizations, and online communities dedicated to specific rare brain disorders. These resources can provide valuable support, information, and connections for individuals and families navigating the challenges of living with or caring for someone with a rare neurological condition.

For health enthusiasts, lifelong learners, and non-specialists, the resources in the appendix can serve as a starting point for further exploration and learning about the fascinating world of rare and mysterious brain disorders. Whether out of curiosity or a desire to deepen their understanding of the human mind, readers from all backgrounds can find valuable information and insights in the resources provided in this section.

11

Glossary of Terms

Adrenoleukodystrophy: A genetic disease that affects the nervous system and adrenal glands, leading to the progressive loss of myelin, the protective sheath that covers nerve fibers.

Agenesis of the Corpus Callosum: A birth defect characterized by the partial or complete absence of the corpus callosum, the band of nerve fibers connecting the two hemispheres of the brain.

Angelman Syndrome: A genetic disorder causing developmental disabilities and nerve-related symptoms, commonly characterized by a happy demeanor, laughter, and smiling.

Anti-NMDA Receptor Encephalitis: An autoimmune disease that occurs when antibodies produced by the body's immune system attack NMDA receptors in the brain, leading to inflammation and a wide range of neurological symptoms.

Capgras Syndrome: A psychological condition where an individual believes that a loved one has been replaced by an impostor. *

*Chiari Malformation:** A condition in which brain tissue extends into the spinal canal, present at birth. It can cause headaches, fatigue, muscle weakness, and other symptoms.

Cotard's Syndrome: A rare disorder in which a person holds a delusional belief that they are dead, do not exist, are putrefying, or have lost their blood or internal organs.

Creutzfeldt-Jakob Disease (CJD): A degenerative brain disorder that leads to dementia and, ultimately, death. It is caused by an abnormal infectious protein called a prion.

Dandy-Walker Syndrome: A congenital brain malformation involving the cerebellum and the fluid-filled spaces around it, often leading to hydrocephalus (fluid accumulation in the brain).

Foreign Accent Syndrome: A rare disorder that causes sufferers to suddenly speak with a perceived foreign accent, often following a brain injury or stroke.

Fragile X Syndrome: A genetic condition that causes a range of developmental problems including learning disabilities and cognitive impairment.

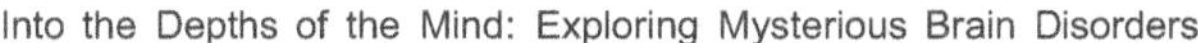

Huntington's Disease: A hereditary, degenerative brain disorder that results in the loss of cognitive, behavioral, and physical control, with symptoms often appearing in mid-adulthood.

Maple Syrup Urine Disease (MSUD): A metabolic disorder characterized by the body's inability to process certain amino acids properly, leading to a sweet-smelling urine, similar to maple syrup, and potential damage to the brain if untreated.

Variant Creutzfeldt-Jakob Disease (vCJD): A type of CJD linked to consuming meat from cattle affected by Bovine Spongiform Encephalopathy (BSE), also known as mad cow disease.

Wilson's Disease (Hepatolenticular Degeneration): A rare genetic disorder that causes excessive copper accumulation in the liver, brain, and other vital organs, leading to hepatic and neurological symptoms.

Neuromyelitis Optica (NMO): Also known as Devic's disease, it is an autoimmune disorder where the immune system attacks the optic nerves and spinal cord, which can lead to vision loss and paralysis.

Neurocysticercosis: A parasitic infection of the nervous system caused by the pork tapeworm. This condition can lead to neurological symptoms when cysts develop within the brain.

Progressive Multifocal Leukoencephalopathy (PML): A rare and often fatal viral disease characterized by progressive damage or inflammation of the white matter of the brain at multiple locations.

Progressive Supranuclear Palsy (PSP): A rare brain disorder that causes serious problems with walking, balance, and eye movements, and can lead to difficulties with swallowing and speaking.

Prion: A type of protein that can trigger normal proteins in the brain to fold abnormally. Prion diseases can affect both humans and animals and are sometimes spread to humans by infected meat products.

Psychosis: A mental disorder characterized by a disconnection from reality, which might manifest as delusions, hallucinations, and impaired thought processes.

Rett Syndrome: A rare, severe neurological disorder that affects the development of the brain, leading to progressive loss of motor skills and speech in young children, especially girls.
 Stiff Person Syndrome (SPS): A neurological disorder with features of an autoimmune disease, SPS is characterized by fluctuating muscle rigidity in the trunk and limbs and a heightened sensitivity to stimuli such as noise, touch, and emotional distress.

12

Index of Disorders

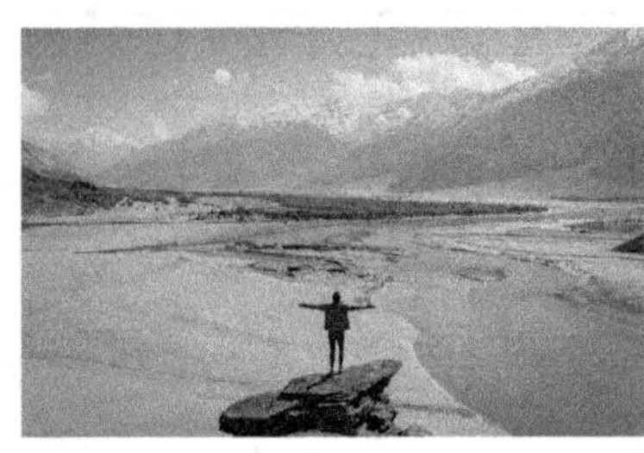

13

Note: This book is intended to provide a comprehensive overview of rare and mysterious brain disorders, featuring case studies, diagnostic criteria, treatment options, and personal stories. It is designed to be accessible to a wide range of audiences, from medical professionals to patients and caregivers, as well as those with a general interest in neuroscience and rare diseases.

"Into the Depths of the Mind: Exploring Mysterious Brain Disorders" is a comprehensive guide aimed at a wide audience interested in delving into the world of rare and mysterious brain disorders. This book features case studies, diagnostic criteria, treatment options, and personal stories to provide a thorough overview of these less-common neurological conditions.

Medical professionals and students, including neurologists, psychiatrists, general physicians, nurses, and medical students, can use this book for reference or to expand their knowledge of rare diseases. Academics and researchers in neuroscience, psychology, or neurological research will also find this collection of rare disorders beneficial for academic and research purposes.

Patients and caregivers seeking detailed information and personal stories for insights and support will also find value in this book. Additionally, medical librarians and institutions looking to enhance their collections with valuable resources for students and researchers may benefit from including this book.

Advocacy groups and NGOs dedicated to supporting individuals with rare brain disorders can utilize this book as an educational resource to inform their work and communities. Health enthusiasts with a general interest in health, medicine, or rare diseases can satisfy their curiosity and deepen their knowledge in this unexplored area. Lifelong learners and non-specialists who enjoy exploring complex topics about the human body and its mysteries will also find this book engaging and informative.

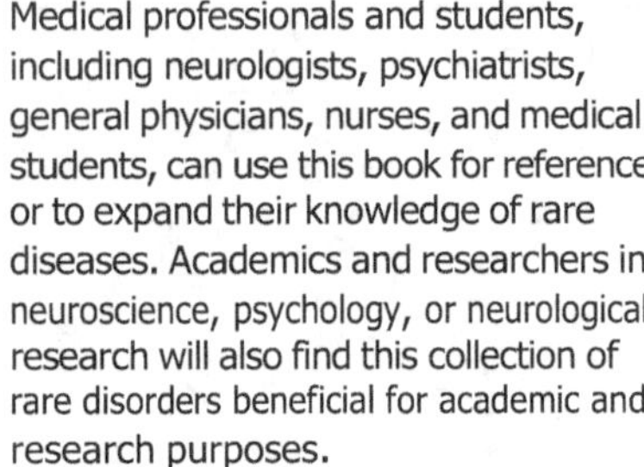

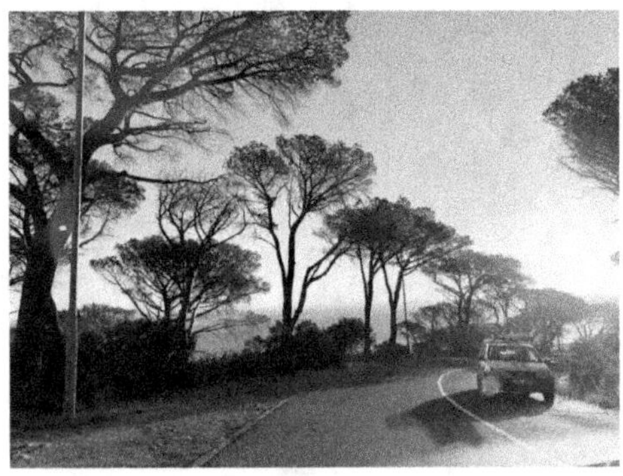

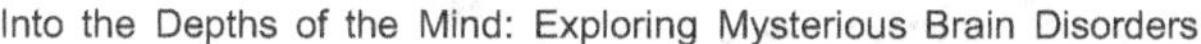

"Minds on the Brink: Unveiling 25 Rare and Mysterious Brain Disorders" offers a unique opportunity to uncover the mysteries of the human mind and gain a deeper understanding of these fascinating conditions."

"Mysteries Within: The Hidden Battles of the Brain"

Dive deep into the enigmatic world of rare neurological disorders with "Mysteries Within: The Hidden Battles of the Brain." Spanning the heartbreaking journey of Rett Syndrome in young girls to the perplexing complexity of diseases like Progressive Supranuclear Palsy, this eye-opening book reveals the struggles, science, and stories behind ten of the most obscure and daunting brain disorders known to medicine. Uncover the bizarre reality of Maple Syrup Urine Disease, where the body's failure to process certain amino acids infuses the urine with a disturbingly sweet scent, signaling deeper dangers for the brain. Encounter the chilling effects of prions with Variant Creutzfeldt-Jakob Disease, the human mirror to mad cow disease, and witness how a misfolded protein can unleash devastation on the human mind. Navigate through the internal storms of neuromyelitis optica, the quiet stealth of neurocysticercosis, and the debilitating stiffness of Stiff Person Syndrome. With profound insights into the labyrinthine pathways of the human nervous system, each page serves as a testimonial to human resilience and our ongoing quest to understand—and ultimately combat—the most cryptic ailments afflicting the brain. As enthralling as it is educational, this book is an essential compass for navigating the lesser-known territories of neurological health and disease.

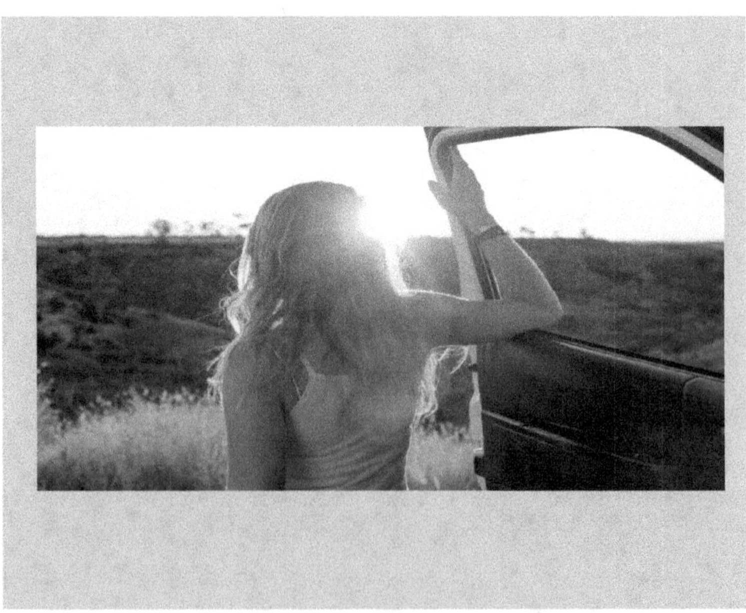

www.ingramcontent.com/pod-product-compliance
Lightning Source LLC
Chambersburg PA
CBHW061252250726
48653CB00002B/626